Praise for Hope Never Dies

"Riveting and richly engrossing stories of courage … never say die."
-Dr. Oz (Mehmet Oz, M.D.)
Host of the Dr. Oz Show and Prof. of Surgery, NYP Columbia Medical Center

"The title says it all. There is no false hope and statistics do not foretell the future. We all have the potential for self-induced healing. There is much to be learned from those who don't die when they are supposed to and both doctors and patients need to be aware of the lessons to be learned."
-Bernie Siegel, M.D.
Author of *Love, Medicine and Miracles* and *The Art of Healing*

"In his outstanding book, ***Hope Never Dies***, Rick Shapiro offers us a window into the lives of extraordinary patients and the paths they have taken to defy the odds of the 'experts'. Through their own stories and the group of practitioners who have provided their unique and different approaches to healing, he provides an inspiration not only for patients and their families, but a critical message for the conventional oncology community to awaken to the value of a true integrative approach that is too frequently absent in cancer care today."
-D. Barry Boyd, M.D., M.S.
Assistant Prof. of Medicine, Yale School of Medicine, Director of Cancer Nutrition, Yale New Haven Health, Senior Attending Medical Oncology, Greenwich Hospital-Yale Health

"Rick Shapiro's amazing book, ***Hope Never Dies***, is a wonderful and important reference for anyone who has been diagnosed with cancer. It is a must read for everyone in the field of oncology, and all my patients, present and future. Read the stories and interviews, digest the material. Your life or that of someone you know may depend on it."
-Robert Zieve, M.D.
Medical Director, Partners in Integrative Cancer Therapies

"Nothing is more powerful than hearing the courageous voices of cancer survivors who chose to take the road less travelled and found themselves thriving. Rick Shapiro has done a masterful job of weaving these survivor stories into a compelling narrative, and the interviews with distinguished cancer doctors add true credibility and inspiration for those who are facing their cancer journey NOW. A must read for anyone who loves someone facing this frightening diagnosis. And that is just about everyone!"
-Helayne Waldman, ED.D., M.S., CNE
Author of *Whole Foods Guide for Breast Cancer Survivors*

"Rick Shapiro's *Hope Never Dies* is an extremely important book. It contains inspiring-patient success stories, along with tremendously informative interviews with five renowned practitioners who have pioneered cutting-edge cancer treatments. The book's twenty cancer patients recount, in their own words, how they were told by their conventional doctors to go home and die—that there were no other options available to them. In each case, through their own efforts, they found integrative and alternative treatments that saved their lives. Their stories are truly riveting. Every person who faces a cancer diagnosis—or who knows someone facing such a diagnosis—should read this book. This means all of us!"
-Julia Schopick, Author of *Honest Medicine*

"What a powerful testament to the strength of the human spirit and the true meaning of hope. The stories of terminal cancer 'thrivers' along with therapies and commentary by leading cancer specialists, makes *Hope Never Dies* a must read for anyone living with cancer, their families, and the medical community at large."
-Tieraona Low Dog, M.D.
Fellowship Director, Academy of Integrative Health and Medicine, and Cancer Thriver

"*Hope Never Dies* is an amazing, empowering book that gives readers a set of invaluable tools to look at a cancer diagnosis through a new and hopeful lens. For the newly diagnosed, or for those already journeying through the labyrinth of cancer, this wonderful book clearly presents integrative medical approaches from some of the leading professionals in the field that will enhance the lives of many."
-Rebecca Katz, M.S.
Author of *The Cancer Fighting Kitchen* and *The Longevity Kitchen*

"*Hope Never Dies* makes three points.
First, some motivated patients far outlive their prognosis, often using integrative cancer treatments. Second, there are some extraordinarily knowledgeable resource people in integrative cancer care. And third, there are critical questions to ask your physician. Integrative cancer care is complex and challenging to get right. Rick Shapiro provides an excellent road map for facing the challenges."
-Michael Lerner, Ph.D.
President and Founder Commonweal, Co-Founder, The Commonweal Cancer Help Program

HOPE
NEVER
DIES

HOW 20
LATE-STAGE AND TERMINAL
CANCER PATIENTS
BEAT THE ODDS

83
Critical Questions
to Ask Before Hiring
Your Cancer
Doctor

INCLUDING

Exclusive Interviews with
5 Renowned Cancer Specialists:
HOW THEY ARE SAVING LIVES NOW

RICK SHAPIRO

Innovative Healing Press

For information about special discounts for bulk purchases please contact:

Innovative Healing Press, LLC
14362 N. Frank Lloyd Wright Boulevard, #73
Scottsdale, Arizona 85260

or

HopeNeverDies.com

Disclaimer:
All content expressed or implied in this book and all related materials is provided for the sole purpose of general educational and informational purposes only. The information is not intended to specify a means of diagnosing, treating, curing, or preventing cancer or any illness. It is not a substitute for treatment by a qualified medical or healthcare professional who should always be consulted before beginning any health program.

Finally, the publisher, author, interviewees, doctors and healthcare practitioners referenced in this book expressly disclaim all responsibility for any liability, loss or risk, personal or otherwise, which is incurred as a consequence, directly or indirectly, from or of the use, effectiveness, safety or application (or lack thereof), of any of the procedures, treatments, therapies or recommendations mentioned, herein.

Designed by GKS Creative, Nashville

Manufactured and Printed in the United States of America.

Library of Congress Control Number: 2017951286

ISBN 978-0-9991997-0-1 (paperback)
ISBN 978-0-9991997-1-8 (e-book)

DEDICATION

To Daniel Shapiro (1917-1996), my father.
He always encouraged me to live life and "go for it."

—and—

To everyone who has faced a cancer diagnosis in the past ...
... and to those who may confront this uninvited intruder in the future.

Rumors of my death are greatly exaggerated.
~Mark Twain

We cannot direct the wind, but we can adjust the sails.
~Anonymous

Courage is not the absence of fear, but rather the judgment that something else is more important than fear.
~Ambrose Redmoon

You gain strength, courage, and confidence by every experience in which you really stop to look fear in the face. You must do the thing which you think you cannot do.
~Eleanor Roosevelt

CONTENTS

"You don't understand. You must face this. You are dying and you
don't have more than a few weeks, maybe 2 months. We don't believe
you will make it until Christmas."
~Diagnosed in 1999

"You have three to four months to live."
~Diagnosed in 2008

"If you don't do chemotherapy and radiation, you will die."
~Diagnosed in 2002

"There are no alternatives. If you don't do chemotherapy, you are insane."
~Diagnosed in 2003

"You have three to six weeks to live."
~Diagnosed in 1995

"If you don't do chemo, you will die."
"If you don't do radiation, you will die."
~Diagnosed in 1993

"You have about two years to live."
~Diagnosed in 1988

AUTHOR'S NOTE

My Evolution Through the Cancer World

On January 15th, 1996, in Phoenix, Arizona, my father's doctor said, "We will bring out the big guns and try to knock this cancer out. It is an aggressive lymphoma, but lymphomas are susceptible to chemotherapy."

After one treatment, my father almost died. The nurses told me they didn't think he would make it through the night as a result of the chemotherapy's effects. We frequently call them "side effects" but their effects can be quite direct.

On February 15th, the same doctor told me, "We look at your Dad's situation as terminal." Just six weeks later, on March 29th, 1996, he was gone. It was a very difficult and sad time.

My Research Begins

In the wake of my father's passing, I wondered why some people afflicted with terminal cancer "beat the odds" and lived many years past their so-called expiration date, while others did not. Were there common denominators prevalent among the unexpected survivors? What distinguished them from the masses?

These issues haunted me. As a result, I developed a strong and resolute desire to find the answers to these questions. In 2001, I began reading numerous books, reports and studies written by doctors, scientists and researchers about conventional, integrative and alternative cancer treatments and therapies.

This thirst for knowledge happened following a health scare I experienced when a highly respected gastroenterologist decided it was prudent to perform a biopsy on my liver. A battery of scans and laboratory tests indicated non-alcoholic fatty liver disease and abnormally high and increasing liver enzyme numbers. I stalled for a bit of time and instead of acquiescing to the biopsy, I made a major transformation in my nutritional habits. My newfound diet was comprised mostly of plant-based food and freshly made veggie juices. I eliminated meat, sugar, confectionary junk, simple carbohydrates and high glycemic foods, thus changing my internal terrain, my biochemistry and, consequently, the health of my liver.

As a result of this major shift, a biopsy was now deemed unnecessary, confirmed by blood tests. This experience awakened me to the power of making major nutritional changes to recover health.

At that time, I also discovered a valuable website known as PubMed, a service of the U.S. National Library of Medicine at the National Institutes of Health (www.ncbi.nim.nih/pubmed). It is comprised of databases that include more than 25 million citations for biomedical literature. Abstracts and full-length text articles regarding diseases, drugs, clinical trials and peer-reviewed studies are part of the millions of documents and literature. It is the world's largest online medical library and an excellent resource of constantly updated information for researchers seeking the latest information about the efficacy of various treatments, chemical agents, natural agents and other therapies.

This site became an incomparable asset, providing me with a wealth of information pertaining to cutting-edge medical studies and literature. I started thinking, "There must be a better way." There must be other treatments and medical options that might be on the frontier or may have been overlooked. I wondered if some of the changes I implemented when dealing with my liver issue could, as part of a more comprehensive and personalized medical protocol, have a material effect on the disease process from a preventative, controlling or eradication standpoint. I became a sponge, absorbing as much medical information as possible; specifically scientific, evidence-based information, recognizing at the same time that dispassionate, rational assessment is always critical.

I wondered, with sorrowful reflection, if my father might be alive if I could have directed him to meaningful, evidence-based research about efficacious integrative or alternative cancer-fighting tools.

Charlatans and Cynics

During my research, I kept in mind that many succumb to the "snake oil pitch" of disingenuous people, especially when facing daunting health challenges. I severely condemn these charlatans who prey upon the fearful and vulnerable with fraudulent promises of miracle cures. Additionally, those naysayers who proactively disparage all integrative and alternative practitioners as quacks also trouble me. Using misinformation and/or disinformation, they often assail effective and safe treatments as voodoo.

Many dismissive accusations are borne out of a lack of knowledge. Other denunciations are premeditated attempts to spread false information about the safety or efficacy of potentially viable treatments. Unfortunately, inflexible detractors often use dogmatic rhetoric to discredit anything out of the norm that does not conform to the conventional and strict "standard of care" as junk science, regardless of credible evidence that may exist to the contrary.

What Constitutes Evidence?

The ambiguous definitions of "evidence" contribute to the huge chasm and disconnect that separates the conventional from the integrative and alternative camps. The conventional establishment does not accept most treatments unless they are blessed by evidence approved by the Food and Drug Administration (FDA). To be blessed, protracted, randomized, large, double blind, placebo-controlled "Phase 3" studies must be conducted. This is the gold standard. These studies cost upwards of one billion dollars. In fact, according to Tufts University Medical School – Study of Drug Development (November 18, 2014), the average pre-tax cost per new prescription drug approval is approximately $2.5 billion. Yes, I said billion with a "B" and it often takes 10 to 15 years to complete—a glacial pace for those who need treatment now. Generally, only large pharmaceutical companies can afford this expense, including the expense of failed, protracted studies. Therefore, if they believe they cannot obtain expedient FDA approvals and financially remunerative patents, they will not pursue such studies or trials.

The integrative and alternative world often uses non-pharmaceutical approaches in their treatment of patients and cannot incur the financial costs of such obscenely expensive studies to validate the efficacy of alternative treatments. They do not have benevolent philanthropists contributing billions of dollars to sponsor protracted research. Consequently, FDA approval is not obtained and the conventional world generally will not recognize such treatments or therapies as acceptable or proven.

Regarding medical studies and published research, Marcia Angell, M.D., a former editor of the *New England Journal of Medicine* (currently, she's a Senior Lecturer in the Department of Global Health and Social Medicine at Harvard Medical School and Faculty Associate with the Center for Bioethics at Harvard Medical School), experienced a close-up perspective of the world of scientific and clinical research for many years. She contends: "Conflicts of interest and biases exist in virtually every field of medicine, particularly those that rely heavily on drugs and devices. It is simply no longer possible to believe much of the clinical research that is published, or rely on the judgment of trusted physicians or authoritative guidelines. I take no pleasure in this conclusion, which I reached slowly and reluctantly over my two decades as an editor of The New England Journal of Medicine."

Personally, I recognize that unbiased and well-designed Phase 3 FDA studies are critically important and that countless studies have engendered efficacious, safe, life-saving drugs. However, I contend that such studies should not necessarily be the only and final arbiter of which treatments and therapies can and should be used to treat patients with cancer.

Unfortunately, the preposterous costs of designing and sponsoring protracted pharmaceutical studies—and the commercial requirement to procure patents to justify these costs—greatly inhibit the probability that non-patentable, non-pharmaceutical agents will ever attract financial sponsors (except on rare occasions), regardless of the potential of producing novel, safe, life-saving treatments for the mass cancer marketplace. Profit motives frequently drive this process.

One must wonder, how many non-patentable, efficacious and safe non-pharmaceutical products and treatments do not reach the marketplace due to the medical system's protracted and expensive approval requirements.

Scientists Taking Risks

I continued my quest to learn about plausible, evidence-based options that might not be prevalent within the conventional medical establishment— options that might be effective in eradicating, controlling or thwarting cancer's grip on people around the world. Recognizing that science is always evolving, and that some of today's unproven treatments may become tomorrow's breakthroughs, we should not forget that some doctors and scientists "on the frontier" are 15 to 25 years ahead of the slow-to-change medical industrial establishment.

One recent example of a doctor, who was ridiculed and then proven correct, stands out. Dan Schectman, Ph.D., an Israeli scientist, was thrown out of his research group in 1982 when he claimed to have discovered a crystalline chemical structure that seemed to violate the laws of nature. In challenging conventional wisdom, he was mocked by his colleagues, but his discovery ultimately altered how chemists conceive of solid matter.

Schectman was vindicated almost 30 years later when he won the Nobel Prize for Chemistry in 2011.

Like Schectman, throughout medical history, many other intrepid doctors and scientists have been ostracized or ridiculed by their colleagues, frequently viewed as crazy and misguided. Likewise, there are many examples of doctors and scientists who were vindicated at later dates and hailed as groundbreakers when their theories were proven correct.

Many doctors and scientists who promote the efficacy of certain integrative and alternative treatments whom I have personally met have also been ridiculed shamelessly. Some of the practitioners I interviewed in Part Two of this book have been chastised because of their unorthodox integrative and alternative treatment practices. However, I believe the preponderance of their methodologies and therapeutic approaches will be accepted universally, at some point, as highly effective-proven contributions to clinical cancer practices, similar to the profound impact engendered by Schectman's groundbreaking contributions in the world of chemistry.

What truly constitutes the concept of "evidence and proof" is open to wide interpretation and debate. This matter is at the heart of the issue of cancer survival for thousands of people who otherwise may be sent down a narrow path of strictly conventional and purportedly "proven" therapies. Too often, these so-called proven therapies do not bring about desired outcomes.

Education and Enlightenment

In March 2010, I attended my first cancer conference. The presentations revolved around the integrative and alternative world of cancer. I went with open-minded skepticism, wanting to hear the voices and opinions of the integrative and alternative camps first-hand.

After sitting through several days of presentations and interacting with highly credentialed doctors and scientists, my interest and focus became more serious. Medical doctors and other cancer specialists from the finest schools told me how they were initially entrenched in conventional practices, but witnessed abysmal outcomes far too frequently. They became disenchanted and sought out other non-conventional treatments and therapies to bring about better results. These doctors had transitioned to a multi-faceted integrative approach.

I also questioned numerous patients; some were in remission, while others were seeking novel, safe and efficacious options to treat their ongoing cancer problems. Much of the information I gleaned, concerning purported effective treatments and therapies, seemed plausible. The conference impelled me to investigate this other realm—integrative and alternative cancer treatments—more deeply.

Since that first cancer conference, I have attended more than twenty conferences nationwide. I have had the privilege of meeting and befriending many highly renowned doctors, scientists, researchers and educators. Based upon my analysis and investigation, I have concluded that many of these people are on the cutting edge, the veritable frontier of new, effective and safe cancer treatments. I have also had the privilege and honor to communicate intimately with hundreds of people whose cancers are in remission or who are actively engaged in fighting this insidious disease. They have invited me in and shared their innermost thoughts, emotions, hopes, and fears, including how they navigated the minefields of treatment options and decisions, and, how the cancer experience has transformed them. Additionally, I have engaged in my own research, evaluating and analyzing hundreds of studies, peer-reviewed medical literature, case studies and other scientific documents concerning all kinds of cancer treatments and therapies.

The remarkable survivor stories in this book confirm the fact that predicting lifespans, even when someone is afflicted with dangerous, biopsy-proven, metastatic cancer, can be erroneous and irresponsible. Unfortunately, many people are inclined to bury their heads under a pillow and go into a deep depression when given a fatalistic prognosis. The concept of hope disappears when they hear a verbal death sentence from their trusted doctor. However, I have found many exceptions—inspiring examples of people living 5, 10 and 20-plus years past their so-called expiration date with a wonderful quality of life.

This book also confirms that there are real options that may be tremendously beneficial, even when people are staring into the abyss, notwithstanding cynical assertions that survivors are just plain lucky or fortunate to have had a spontaneous remission. It is my contention that these people are alive due to rational, evidence-based medical interventions—and not due to luck or spontaneous remission.

In fact, I believe the term spontaneous remission is a misnomer and should be renamed "rational remission," as there is bountiful evidence of integrative and alternative treatments and therapies that have a "rational" scientific basis for changing one's internal bio-chemical status and/or arresting cancer progression, which may bring about unexpected remissions.

In my research, I found a powerful and revealing book. In 1993, the Institute of Noetic Sciences published *Spontaneous Remission: An Annotated Bibliography*, by Caryle Hirshberg and Brendan O'Regan. This telling publication provides details of over 3,500 cases of spontaneous remission, derived from 800 journals in 20 different countries. The book's authors suggest that there are many underreported cases of spontaneous remission, and that research has shown that the number of actual spontaneous remission cases has been on the increase.

Let me be clear. I do not believe that there are any singular magic elixirs, nor formulaic recipes for beating cancer. This book does not endorse any particular treatment as a panacea nor does it claim that any particular doctor or clinic has the omniscient ability to cure cancer. However, the plethora of astonishing life-saving outcomes documented herein strongly suggests that there are compelling options that should be closely investigated and, when appropriate, implemented as part of a well-conceived, comprehensive and carefully tailored cancer strategy.

Although the number of my interviews does not constitute a large sample, my personal research and experience clearly shows that these survivors are a microcosm of thousands who have beaten the odds (after being told there was no hope) by implementing evidence-based, integrative, and alternative therapeutic strategies.

It should be noted that most people explore integrative and alternative treatments as a last resort, after strict conventional treatments have failed. Think about how outcomes might be positively impacted if safe, efficacious integrative or alternative treatments were implemented early on—when people are first diagnosed versus after having been subjected to harsh therapies which may seriously impact one's vitality, immune system and ability to fight or control cancer.

Research, Compare, Contemplate—Then Act

This book is meant to empower, galvanize and stimulate people to consider thinking outside the box—or even expand the box—concerning personalized oncology medicine, so that cancer patients may become more knowledgeable about efficacious and safe options that are not recognized within the prevalent convention known as "standard of care." It is also meant to open skeptical and cynical minds to contemplate new possibilities and paths worthy of consideration.

I am here to apprise you that many other proven options exist. With the help of knowledgeable, scientifically sophisticated integrative and alternative healthcare practitioners, they are available for your consideration.

Please note, it is not my intention to stoke the flames of medical controversy, in fact it is quite the opposite. I fully acknowledge that there are many conventional treatments regarding all kinds of health conditions—including cancer—which save lives on a daily basis. This book, however, is intended to provide hope, inform and encourage you to ask important questions; to spur you to consider the importance of potential integrative and alternative treatments and therapies. I believe it would be profoundly constructive and rational for the clinical and scientific pundits of the different camps to engage in open, continuing and honest dialogue to bring about a greater understanding of the collaborative strengths of safe and effective non-conventional treatments combined with safe and effective conventional treatments. A concerted effort to combine the medical intellect of the respective leaders of all points of view could ultimately bring about much improved outcomes for innumerable cancer patients worldwide.

It is my deepest hope that readers of this book will take a few moments and reflect before embarking upon the daunting journey of choosing a cancer strategy. I hope it will help those who are paralyzed with fear to conjure up the courage to find the wisdom to make fully informed and well-reasoned decisions prior to leaping impulsively into any cancer protocol or regimen; to become critical thinkers, not cynical critics in the quest to ultimately find peace, enduring health and a greater quality of life.

Godspeed and Keep the Hope!
Rick Shapiro

PART ONE

How 20 Late-Stage and Terminal Cancer Patients Beat the Odds

About Part One The following true stories chronicle the journeys of 20 people who were given a dire cancer prognosis. Their stories are candid, enlightening and heartfelt. They provide unique insights from personal and medical perspectives. I interviewed all of them myself.

They are remarkable accounts of courageous people who survived terrible prognoses—and all of them continue to thrive today. Some were given as little as three weeks to live; most were told they would die within one year. All of them, as of the date of this publication, are thriving and have outlived their prognoses by 5 to 25+ years. At the beginning of each chapter, notice their dates of diagnosis and the dire comments of many of their doctors.

These stories are their stories. There are no guarantees that the different paths taken to wellness will prove to be beneficial to anyone else. Everyone is an individual and everyone possesses his or her own unique medical fingerprint and biochemical status. Therefore, the effects of different treatments and therapies can vary from person to person, regardless if two people have been diagnosed with the same cancer and the same stage of such cancer or not.

Of the 20 people I interviewed, 19 are identified with their real names. Only one person shall remain anonymous, and that person is specified as such in his chapter.

Book Format Most of this book is composed of the words spoken by cancer patients and doctors transcribed from my personal interviews with them. Each patient's dialogue follows his or her introduction with the word "Meet." My comments are in this **san serif** font; the stories they tell in their own words are in a serifed font. And, when emphasis is necessary, you'll see their comments in ***bold italic font***.

ELIZABETH

Elizabeth Panke, Ph.D., M.D.
Ovarian Cancer
Diagnosed in 1999

"You don't understand, you must face this; you are dying.
You don't have more than a few weeks, maybe two months.
We don't believe you will make it until Christmas."
~Medical doctors and social workers at cancer treatment centers,
nationwide, where Dr. Panke went for treatment

Her Early Years Elizabeth Panke was born in Poland in 1950. She was fascinated with and immersed herself in science, even as a child. At age 14, she immigrated to the U.S.

Elizabeth majored in chemistry in college, obtained a master's degree from the University of Southern California in physical therapy, a Ph.D. in experimental pathology and a medical degree from the University of Cincinnati College of Medicine. She also completed an anatomic and clinical pathology residency and a fellowship in molecular biology, spending over four years at the University of Cincinnati. Her academic, clinical, scientific and medical credentials are exemplary.

In 1988, Elizabeth founded and developed a DNA laboratory that evolved into an enterprise known as Genetica DNA Laboratory in Cincinnati. Elizabeth became a known expert and leader in the field of DNA identity, parentage and biological family relationship testing. Under her direction, the lab earned a very strong national and international reputation.

She led a busy, hectic life, managing and leading Genetica, lecturing at numerous conferences around the U.S., authoring scientific articles, acting as an expert witness, and raising a family.

Shocking Discovery In June of 1999, during a routine gynecological examination, Elizabeth's doctor discovered the existence of minor irregular bleeding. She was only 49 years old. During the last week of June, Elizabeth underwent an ultrasound and a large tumor was found on her ovary. On July 6th, her doctor informed her that she had Stage 3 ovarian and uterine cancer, which had now spread to the abdomen.

Meet Elizabeth

I was shocked. I had no family history of cancer. I was so angry. Why and how did this happen to me? One week after my diagnosis, a surgeon removed my ovaries, my uterus and any visible cancer. I went on chemo two weeks after the surgery.

Standard of Care: Chemotherapy

Although I was a very experienced doctor with a deep scientific and medical background, I did not question my doctor.

> **I went with the standard chemotherapy for my type of cancer. They said the chemo would probably take care of the problem, despite the micro-metastases.**

They said there was better than a 50 percent chance that I would go into long-term remission. I lost all my hair, bought a wig, was getting Taxol and Carboplatin, took nausea medication, continued to work and pushed on. The experience was quite strenuous. I started treatments in the middle of July and ended toward the end of August 1999. Honestly, I felt quite lousy.

Unfortunately, my cancer was very happy; it grew very aggressively during this time. I had so many malignant ascites. My microscopic tumors were growing rapidly. It seemed like the chemo was feeding the tumors in my abdomen. I also had developed a tumor in my spleen. The chemo did not work; in fact a gallon of malignant fluid was pulled out of my abdomen every five days.

Chemo Did Not Work: If at First You Don't Succeed, Try, Try Again

At this point, recognizing that the chemo was not helping, they tried another chemo drug. After several weeks on the new chemo drug combination, nothing good happened. I was losing all of my white blood cells and needed shots to help my bone marrow work! The doctors then said, "We must try something different."

I asked, "What are we going to try? We have had two failures; if the next effort fails, I won't have much left. Let's get some outside opinions from various experts."

> **I was going down fast. My doctors were not interested in outside opinions, so I decided I needed to take matters into my own hands.**

I traveled to five very prestigious cancer centers throughout the United States, including major centers in New York, Texas and California. I received various recommendations. One doctor told me to go with a higher dose of the same chemo I had been taking, but that would require a bone marrow transplant, which I felt could easily kill me.

Another doctor said, "Do a high dose irradiation of the abdominal area," but I felt this might be like a death sentence. They had no idea at all if their suggestions would have any impact or if I would survive more grueling treatments. They did not know what to do. I had metastatic cancer; two different kinds of chemotherapy did not work and the cancer was spreading.

At this point, several of the cancer center doctors sat me down in October of 1999 and told me that I needed to face reality; that it was doubtful that I would make it until Christmas. I was in disbelief, angry, upset and desperate.

Chemosensitivity Testing

I had heard of chemosensitivity testing, but did not know much about it. Essentially, this is a laboratory testing procedure where a cancer patient's actual malignancy or tissue sample is exposed to different chemotherapy drugs, one at a time and in different chemo combinations, to assess sensitivity and responses. You can't get any more personal or customized in testing methodology than that.

I inquired and was told by all of the cancer institutions that it did not work. Yet, I needed to take action, immediately. I was dying and had no time to waste.

I had heard of a particular laboratory in Southern California. I sent them a sample of my ascites. They tested my sample against a variety of chemotherapy cocktails and concluded that Taxol and Carboplatin would work. I knew without question they were wrong, because I had already tried that combination and it had failed.

Internet Research and Robert Nagourney, M.D.

I was not giving up, so I searched the Internet day and night trying to find hope, a treatment, someone who could help me. I came across Dr. Robert Nagourney's website. Dr. Nagourney is a medical doctor, a practicing oncologist who also owns and operates a chemosensitivity laboratory known as Rational Therapeutics in Long Beach, California. In reading about his lab, I noticed a material difference between his lab and the lab with people who said Taxol and Carboplatin would work. I noticed that his lab personnel did their testing quite differently from the other lab's methodology.

I called Dr. Nagourney the next day, got him on the phone, and was very impressed with his opinions, explanations and research. He sounded very logical as we discussed his work, patient outcomes, and the science substantiating his opinions. I immediately investigated everything he said, and then decided to send Dr. Nagourney a fresh sample of my ascites.

Dr. Nagourney sounded very positive on the phone. He treated me like a human being. He gave me hope.

Within a few days, Dr. Nagourney called me and said, "I have a combination that is making the cancer cells just melt away." The combination was Gemzar and Platinol. This was a chemotherapy combination that no other medical oncologist from any cancer center had recommended.

I jumped on an airplane the next morning and saw Dr. Nagourney that very same day. He drew malignant cells from my abdomen, and then injected the chemo directly into my abdomen, directly at the tumors. He wanted direct, undiluted contact. No one else had recommended this procedure. I was anxious, but hopeful. He also injected the personalized chemotherapy cocktail, derived specifically from the results of the lab test on my ascites, into my vein.

Then, for my second treatment, he drew the fluid out, only about a quart, not a gallon. Under the microscope it looked like the malignant cells were beat up. After the second treatment, which was just three weeks into my chemo treatment, there was no more fluid to withdraw.

By Christmas, there was no evidence of any more malignant cells in my body. I was supposed to be dead by Christmas, but instead, my cancer cells were dead! This was after six cycles of Dr. Nagourney's chemotherapy. No evidence of cancer, as confirmed by CT scan, PET scan, ultrasound, and, physical exam.

Dr. Nagourney said, "We can't see it, but you must have a microscopic disease." He encouraged me to continue chemo treatments until May of 2000, at which time I had surgery to explore the area to see if there was any more evidence of cancer.

The surgeons took several biopsies during the surgery; however, pathological exams indicated everything was clean. Dr. Nagourney prudently recommended that I continue treatments, once per month, for a year, to kill any microscopic disease. To this day, every six months, I have my blood checked for tumor markers and I get an annual physical.

Conventional Institutional Opinions: "You are lucky ..."
Conventional institutions gave no credibility to Dr. Nagourney's treatments. They assumed his treatments were not credible, because they assumed incorrectly that he used old testing methodologies, not the newer methodologies that Dr. Nagourney employs in his laboratory tests. They don't care, nor do they want to understand why or how I happen to be here, in the flesh. It is sad and so disappointing.

> **I informed the major cancer centers that I had visited and consulted with of my wonderful outcome, the fact that the cancer was gone. To my dismay, all they had to say was, "You are lucky."**

In my opinion, Dr. Nagourney is brilliant! I absolutely believe, without question, I am only alive because I came across Dr. Nagourney's website. Today, the chemotherapy combination used on me by Dr. Nagourney has become an internationally recognized and widely used combination.

When people hear my story and call me, I would say only 50 percent of the patients pursue the possibility of going down this road with their doctors.

Unfortunately, most of their doctors talk them out of getting tested in this manner. They either tell their patients, "This is the drug we use for your type of cancer," or "We do our own type of chemosensitivity testing."

However, their testing methodology is far different from Dr. Nagourney's. They are night-and-day different! Even if 25 percent of the people I talk with on the phone agree to go forward with Dr. Nagourney's test, many of these patients' oncologists will not follow the suggested regimen. Sometimes patients must change doctors to get the treatment recommended by him.

Transformation and Pearls of Wisdom
In the beginning of this journey, I felt disbelief and anger. Since my successful treatments, I came to accept 'what is' and enjoy 'the moments in life.' I don't have all the answers. My role is to do the best I can

in my life, moment-to-moment. I don't know if I am cured, but it has now been 17 years.

Once a year, my husband and I fly to Los Angeles to help raise funds for the Vanguard Foundation. This is a non-profit founded by Dr. Nagourney to help people who cannot afford to pay for the test. Unfortunately, insurance does not pay for it. It is looked at by the insurance companies as experimental, at best.

I have also started a foundation in Cincinnati, which I funded with $100,000, to help people who cannot afford the test in my metropolitan area. I try to get the word out in the community. Again, I feel I am alive because I stumbled onto his website.

It is sad, but I find that some cancer patients are not sure if they want to live. You must want to live. I find that cancer patients who do the best are those who become advocates for themselves, who direct their own therapies versus patients who just go along with their doctors.

They should not be afraid of innovative treatments versus the old conventional therapies.

There is one other doctor in addition to Dr. Nagourney who is also involved in this cutting-edge testing methodology: Dr. Larry Weisenthal, also of Southern California. They are former partners, and the two of them are the best, anywhere. Regarding my desire to inform people about the test and Dr. Nagourney, I will talk to anyone, anytime, day or night.

People should not lose hope. Keep on searching; follow your heart.

JULIE

Julie Zahniser
Breast Cancer
Diagnosed in 2008

"You have three to four months to live."
~Doctor's prognosis

Her Early Years Growing up, Julie was a fun loving, happy-go-lucky kid. Born in an upper middle class neighborhood in Miami, Florida, she enjoyed a stable, normal upbringing. She was an excellent student and even a better sailor, a national championship sailor and board surfer, competing all over the U.S. and the world. She was such an elite and successful competitor that she was recruited to race as a member of the Junior Olympic Sailing Team.

Upon graduating from high school, Julie continued her passion for sailing at Dartmouth College, where she ultimately became captain of the team. After graduating in 1988 with a degree in Government, she ventured west to attend law school at UCLA. Upon graduation she worked for a regional law firm and subsequently set up her own law practice back in Fort Pierce, Florida. In 2002, Julie married Adam. Soon thereafter, in 2004, her family grew with the addition of beautiful twin daughters, Caroline and Kimberly.

Life was good, smooth sailing in all quarters...until....

Unusual Warning Signs One morning in May of 2007, Julie awoke with a strong premonition. She never felt she possessed clairvoyant or visionary powers, but unmistakably, an inner intuition spoke to her and said, "You have cancer."

There was no rational basis for this startling epiphany, but it continued on and on, causing Julie continuous anxiety. It pervaded her thoughts day and night, so she finally went to a hypnotherapist for the first time in her life. She needed to expunge this haunting feeling. The strong feelings stayed with Julie, despite the absence of any discomfort, pain or atypical manifestations of anything abnormal. The hypnotherapist was unable to assuage her anxiety.

Her angst continued unabated, so she went to see another hypnotherapist, but the inner voice telling her she had cancer did not subside. This hypnotherapist strongly suggested she see a medical doctor. She visited several conventional and alternative practitioners. However, she says, "They all brushed me off." They felt she was paranoid. With the absence of any symptoms, they refrained from performing any scans, lab work, or tests to assess whether she had any signs of cancer.

A Poor Prognosis: Triple Negative Breast Cancer One year later, in May of 2008, Julie felt a lump, essentially a large lymph node. She proceeded to visit a conventional and alternative doctor, both of whom said that it was probably nothing. They both told her to wait six to eight weeks and come back if it was still there.

The lump did not abate and Julie could not wait any longer. Five weeks later she went back to her primary doctor, who sent her for a surgical consult. After a mammogram showed tangible evidence of probable cancer involvement with nine lymph nodes, Julie underwent an excisional biopsy.

On May 20th, 2008, upon receiving her pathology report, Julie was told she had a very aggressive, triple negative breast cancer, 9 of 9 lymph nodes involved, indicating a poor prognosis.

Meet Julie

It is somewhat crazy to see a doctor and say, "I think I have cancer." The doctor said, "The cancer has metastasized, but we have very good support groups." Not exactly comforting or optimistic words.

> **The pathologist told me she had never seen**
> **any breast cancer that was this aggressive.**
> **Tears were flowing down my face.**

After the biopsy, Julie chose to see a different doctor for a lumpectomy. Her new doctor performed an axillary dissection and removed 36 lymph nodes. To make matters worse, after her pathology report came back, the surgeon told her she should have chemo and radiation. Without it, she was told, she could expect to live approximately three to four months, but he indicated quite strongly that even with treatment there was not much hope.

Julie was not interested in hearing predictions of her lifespan, but it was too late. The doctor spilled this mind-numbing news without asking her if she wanted to know about her statistical prognosis.

> **The news was devastating. I was thinking**
> **of my 4-year-old twins who needed me.**
> **I wanted to see them grow up.**

Was Julie's premonition, a year hence, a coincidence, or unexplainably yet remarkably prophetic? Whatever the essence of her previous intuition, unmistakably, Julie had a very dangerous and potentially lethal prognosis.

Prognosis Based on "Standard of Care," but Mom's Experience Enlightened Me

My doctor said, "Try to get into a clinical trial at a major cancer center." That is code for, "There is not much hope."

I realized that percentages and time frames are based on standard of care protocols, which represent the overwhelming number of conventional treatments offered in the U.S. and worldwide. The key phrase here is *standard of care*, because standard of care does not include unconventional or alternative treatments, nor does it take into account the individual. It is based on broad-based statistics involving thousands and thousands of people.

Standard of care involves surgery, chemotherapy and radiation, not integrative or alternative options.

I had an advantage that many people don't have. My mom died of lung cancer five years before, and during her experience with Stage 3b lung cancer, I did a huge amount of research. I spent thousands of hours reading virtually every abstract from clinical studies that I could find. I traveled with her to major cancer centers in Texas and Chicago to investigate clinical trials. The data did not speak to hope and positive outcomes.

I learned, as a result of my research, that chemo drugs frequently only give you several extra months to live. The studies do not speak in terms of years; survival benefit is measured in terms of months. For me, I knew there were possible alternatives beyond standard of care, though I had moments of real doubt.

**At times I asked myself, "Do I really want to survive?"
because I felt it might be easier to go along with what
the doctors told me to do. Frequently, it is easier
to go along with the herd.**

The decision of Julie's path soon became obvious to her. The doctors were pessimistic and offered nothing beyond treatments from their conventional toolbox: chemo and radiation.

They were very pessimistic to begin with, and my own research confirmed their dire prognosis. I wanted to live and did not have faith in chemo and radiation. I decided to fight and knew I needed to know as much as the doctors, and not let other people make these life and death decisions, but doubts lingered. How could the whole medical world be wrong? Was I fooling myself against all hope that I could beat the odds?

Finding Hope Across the Atlantic

Julie knew she would have to search for treatments or therapies beyond the scope of the conventional standard of care.

I wanted the cutting edge of medicine; I wanted to look outside the box.

I found that you can't get that at the major U.S. cancer centers.

While searching the Internet, voraciously, day and night, only one month after my diagnosis, I came across a documentary by a cancer researcher named Burton Goldberg. In the documentary, he talked of integrative treatments offered in Germany that were more progressive than anything offered in the U.S.

One of the doctors in the documentary, Ursula Jacob, spoke about cancer therapies and the need to eradicate micro-metastases at the cellular level. Her words resonated with me. I knew from my research for my mom, there had been some positive results with vaccine therapy in clinical trials in the U.S., but I couldn't get into any relevant trials. I also discovered that they were doing vaccine therapy and many progressive treatments in Germany not found in the U.S.

After a couple of phone calls with Dr. Jacob and a huge leap of faith, 10 days after viewing the documentary, I was on a flight to Germany to meet with the one doctor who gave me some semblance of hope. I needed to move quickly.

Upon arriving in Germany, under Dr. Jacob's guidance, I underwent a battery of tests. She conducted a Circulating Tumor Cell (CTC) test, among other tests. She did not sugarcoat my prognosis and told me that because of the cancer's aggressiveness I had a poor prognosis, but she never wavered in her feeling that I had a real chance. She knew I had a great will to live.

I was in relatively good shape, cancer aside, and desperately wanted to see my daughters grow up. I was willing to be disciplined in working closely and confidently with her. She also knew I had the unwavering support of Adam, my husband, who was with me every step of the way, and who accompanied me to Germany.

Multiple Treatments and Therapies

I received many different treatments and therapies during my five visits to Germany. I went every three to four months for a year and a half. The treatments varied during each trip. I was constantly monitored with PET scans and CTC tests. The treatments included:

1. Low dose chemotherapy based on CTC tests, during the first three visits
2. Several vaccines (dendritic autologuous vaccines)
3. Different thymus extracts (injections)
4. Various peptides
5. Anti-viral treatments
6. Hyperthermia treatments
7. Lots of herbs and other supplements, by injection and orally, (approximately 60-70 supplements orally) per day
8. Mistletoe injections
9. High dose intravenous vitamin C
10. Quercetin
11. Iodine treatments, and other treatments as well

The "standard of care" chemo treatments would not have worked for me, according to the chemosensitivity tests I had in Germany. It is important to get it right on the first try or you needlessly go through difficult, often debilitating chemotherapy regimens for nothing.

When I had chemotherapy, I had virtually no side effects. I believe this is due to the other treatments, including specific herbs I took simultaneously when receiving my chemo treatments. They reduced the potential toxicity tremendously.

Conventional protocols are not too effective with advanced cancer, and they are so hard on people.

Progress

My CTC tests started out with scary, astronomically high numbers. Ideally, you want to be under 5.0 and closer to 1.0, but I started out at 2,000. After a variety of treatments over the course of my visits to Germany, my numbers declined to 13.8, still very high, but moving in the right direction, then to 6.0 and then to 3.0.

Dr. Jacob preferred to use a laboratory in Greece for her work. A similar test in the U.S. is called the Cellsearch CTC. I also had this test performed in the U.S. at Quest. It indicated an optimum 0.0 number; fantastic results. I thought Dr. Jacob's methodology was ingenious, the way she changed up the treatment protocols at every visit to keep the cancer off guard.

Whenever I returned to Florida, between visits to Germany, I worked with an alternative doctor and continued with high dose intravenous vitamin C twice per week. I also ingested 60-70 specific supplements per day, to strengthen my immune system.

Mind-Body and Dealing with Fear

I should mention that throughout my treatments, I did yoga, meditation, and visualization, and listened to the Kelly Howell Brain Think CDs. These mind-body treatments were very helpful. I was very fearful during the process.

I was not only fearful, I was fearing the fear!

What finally worked for me was not trying to make the fear go away, but trying to observe the fear and to say, "Oh, you are here today," and not pressuring myself to conquer it.

Taking Care of Myself

The last trip I made to Germany was in late 2009. I correspond with Dr. Jacob regularly and continue to get CTC tests and PET scans here in Florida. I have cleaned up our water system at home and rid our house of all toxins. Cancer made me focus on my health. I eat 100 percent organically now and only eat grass-fed meat and wild salmon, when eating animal products. I still get vitamin C infusions and have reduced my supplements to approximately 15 per day.

I feel wonderful, better now than I did before I had cancer. I exercise constantly and am happy! If my cancer recurs, we will catch it early and I believe we will be able to handle it.

During my treatments with Dr. Jacob, I looked at her as 'the conductor;' however, I was a very active participant. I believe she saved my life, but it was my own research, and putting together a proactive team that played a huge role in allowing me to be here today. I had a hormone doctor, an alternative doctor, another alternative doctor whom I consulted, an oncologist for insurance reasons and foremost, Dr. Jacob.

Some treatments were automatically covered by insurance, but I also hired a company to submit my German insurance claims. This company was paid on a contingency basis. Cancer treatments are very expensive, but I decided not to worry about the money.

This was my life and nothing was more important than my health, for me, my husband and my children.

Transformation and Pearls of Wisdom

I have gained a tremendous appreciation for every day I am alive. I looked down the barrel of a gun. My transformation has been immensely positive. Life is just beautiful. Enjoy it!

If you are considering conventional treatments, take a close look at the success of those treatments. Don't blindly follow the herd.

HOLLIE

Hollie Quinn
Breast Cancer
Diagnosed in 2002

"If you don't do chemotherapy and radiation, you will die."
~Doctor's prognosis

Her Early Years Hollie grew up in an affluent, happy household in Los Angeles. Although her childhood was easy and carefree, she did get sick quite often. She had tuberculosis as a young child and due to a variety of maladies, including gastrointestinal issues, migraines, allergies and vertigo, she was subjected to many x-rays.

Hollie received her undergraduate degree from the University of California at Santa Barbara in 1996 and, subsequently, a master's degree in Public Policy from the University of Chicago in 1998. Shortly after graduation, she married her sweetheart, Patrick, whom she met in graduate school. One year later, the happy couple moved to Los Angeles. It was a blissful time. The young couple was excited about the future and very much in love.

Discovery and Terror In August of 2002, the happy couple was expecting the birth of their first child in just two weeks. It was an exciting time! One Sunday night, Hollie was relaxing at home watching television and her hand brushed up against her breast where she felt a lump. She had never felt anything like this and became sick to her stomach. She went to her doctor the next day, had a biopsy and then encountered the longest 48 hours of her life while awaiting the test results.

Three days had elapsed since feeling the lump, and when Hollie arrived home after shopping, there was a voicemail from her doctor: "Give me a call and tell the nurse to interrupt me when you call."

She called immediately and the doctor said, "The tests came back malignant."

Hollie was "numb, terrified, and in shock." She was 27 years old, 38 weeks pregnant, and just two weeks from delivering her first child.

Meet Hollie

Despite my emotional, crying state, I knew I needed to move forward. I went to the doctor's office with Patrick to check the baby's health, but couldn't do any more testing of the cancer since my baby was 38 weeks along. That night, I went to the hospital to get induced and gave birth the next morning.

I had no knowledge about cancer, or integrative or alternative medicine. I only knew of conventional medicine. 'Was there any other kind?'

With my cancer, we were on a fast track. One week later I had surgery; a lumpectomy to remove the cancer. It was Stage 2. We (my husband and I) were just following orders. If my doctor said we needed to do something, we just did it; we did not think about it. Who was I to question these doctors?

After my surgery, we started to do research about what we should do. We both had backgrounds as trained social scientists and knew how to engage in analytical thinking. My doctors said I needed to do aggressive radiation and chemotherapy, then five years of hormonal therapy, specifically Tamoxifen.

This, in itself, was terrifying. Something deep inside of me hesitated.

My intuition said, "No, you should not do these treatments." I was now the young mother of a healthy baby girl.

We put on our analytical hats and engaged in more research; we questioned the effectiveness of these treatments. I asked my doctors lots of questions and suggested that these treatments might not be the best regimen for me. I read everything I could get my hands on from the bookstore and the Internet. I wanted to know as much about the treatments as the doctors.

I asked the doctors about success rates. I was told there was a "10 percent reduced recurrence" for people like me, based on some studies. But, what does "10 percent reduced recurrence" mean when you are 27 years old, and your body has just gone through the transformations associated with giving birth to your first child? Ten percent reduced from what? Patrick found a study that suggested radiation reduced local recurrences, but radiation was not helpful in improving survival.

We were still at a loss, trying to figure out what to do. I did not want to do nothing, but the conventional therapies did not appear promising, given the probable consequences. I went to a number of doctors seeking answers and direction, armed with my notepad and 30 questions. Some doctors were patient; others were not. Some said, "Why are you asking these questions?" "Why are you thinking about this?" "You need to do chemo."

Then, serendipity struck. After telling a neighbor of my dilemma, he recommended I see a local Asian doctor who only worked with supplements. I made an appointment and visited this doctor who patiently explained how and why supplements could have such a powerful effect. At this first meeting, the doctor pulled a book off her bookshelf by Donald Yance. The doctor said, "This guy knows what he is talking about. Read it."

I went home and read the entire book that night, and this was no small book. I called Donald Yance's office, also known as the Mederi Foundation, the next morning, but found out he was booked two months in advance.

At the Precipice

I was now less than one week from the beginning of my scheduled chemo-therapy treatments. Despite my independent research, the momentum toward beginning my scheduled treatments was overwhelming. My family and friends were supportive, but they encouraged the conventional path. The doctors said we must go with conventional treatments, that there were no other options. Patrick noticed the prognostic indicators in the pathology report appeared less than optimistic. The word "unfavorable" was strewn throughout the report.

I arranged a phone consultation with Donald Yance's office. They pushed me to stall the chemo treatments one week, because his office needed time to review the medical information I submitted. They also needed time to evaluate the additional tests I underwent for them, more specific blood work testing a variety of things that conventional medicine does not recognize.

I talked to a woman named Chancal Cabrera, my contact at Mederi. She said I needed to stabilize my body, that I just had a baby and my body was not yet in its best, healthiest state for chemo. She was not a proponent of chemo, but indicated strongly, that if I were to pursue chemo, the time was not right. At the same time, my conventional doctors did not feel that my baby's recent birth was relevant in any way to whether I had chemo treatments now or later.

> Hollie was facing enormous pressure: family and peer pressures, the issue of whether or not to follow a conventional path strongly recommended by respected doctors, or to follow some exotic, foreign concept known as botanical-herbal medicine. Everything was at stake: her health, her family's future, and her very survival.

Finally, after talking to Chancal and the people at Mederi, I made my mind up. I would not go down the conventional path. Not because I was grasping at alternative pathways, but because I felt the research strongly indicated, logically, that the conventional path and past studies did not show very favorable results.

**On the other hand, the botanical path made more sense
to me. It seemed logical, it was non-toxic
and my research indicated that it brought about
much more favorable results.**

Once I made my decision I was optimistic and excited. Now, I had to tell my doctor my decision. This was not easy. Doctors are supposed to know what to do. We are supposed to trust their wisdom and recommendations. When I told my doctor, he responded, "If you don't do chemo and radiation, you will die."

Another doctor was compassionate and tried to talk me into radiation, but we rejected this suggestion, because radiation did not correlate with greater survival. Some doctors never talked to us again; they treated us disrespectfully. Some of my friends and family were also very critical. They took the position that the botanical-herbal medicine must be bogus or it would be commonplace.

Looking back, my fear about the treatment was greater than my fear about the cancer.

Herbal Medicine Treatment and Side Effects Hollie's protocol was comprised of taking approximately 70 to 80 different pills per day. Many different supplements, including vitamins, botanicals and other herbal formulations made up the bulk of her regimen. Specific smoothie formulations, tinctures and teas were also strongly recommended. Exercise, eating specific healthy foods, avoiding other foods and incorporating a mind-body approach was critical as well. Every recommendation had a purpose. Abundant scientific, evidence-based studies created the foundation for everything the Mederi Foundation recommended for Hollie's protocol.

The side effects of her protocol brought about a quizzical yet wonderful result, as Patrick excitedly pointed out: "When the protocol started to kick in, Hollie had a whole cascade of collateral health benefits. Her vertigo went away, her migraines disappeared, and her gastrointestinal problems went away. The protocol not only dealt with her cancer, but also improved her health and immunity, on many fronts, which strengthened her immune system and many internal health systems. The conventional doctors had no interest in knowing what Hollie was doing. Occasionally, they would ask, 'How is that diet thing going?'"

Every six weeks, Hollie had blood work that she sent to the people at Mederi to evaluate her health. The results of these lab reports provided Mederi with continual information that engendered adjustments to her dosage and continual tweaking of her supplementation and diet.

At the same time, Hollie underwent exams by an open-minded oncologist every six weeks. She took nothing for granted, and also had imaging tests every six months. The oncologist checked tumor markers, but would not order certain other tests we requested, recommended by Mederi, because the oncologist felt they were meaningless and irrelevant.

Doctors are 'type A people;' egocentric and smart. It is easier for them to dismiss me as lucky than to look into whether their recommendations are wrong. There is tremendous money behind chemo and other drugs. I am told they can lose their medical license if they recommend something like botanical medicine.

Unfortunately, the products recommended in my protocol are not paid for by insurance. This is a sad state of affairs. The first month, my products cost around $1,000 and then $700 to $900 a month; approximately 70 to 80 pills per day and occasional phone consultations. This is all out of pocket.

We transformed our lifestyle, threw out all bad food, personal care products, cleaning products, and anything that might be toxic. There is a lot you can control.

Generally, all of our food is organic, whole foods, not processed, and we eat very little meat or poultry. We eat lots of vegetables. I was on the original protocol for three years, every day. After three years, I went on a maintenance protocol where I cut back my pills approximately 50 percent. A high percentage of recurrences happen in the first two years. After two years my fears began to subside, and after five years another great leap forward occurred with the arrival of my second daughter.

> **The best doctors in Los Angeles said I needed to go down the conventional path. How many other women go down this fear-based road? People are quick to judge when they have not walked in your shoes. The issues are not black and white.**

Some of our friends made lifestyle changes after seeing how and what I did. Some just think, "You are lucky." As a result of my experience, our lifestyles have changed entirely. We seek naturopathic medicine for ourselves and the kids. We take nothing for granted. Cancer puts things into perspective. Nothing is too challenging for us. During the past five years, we have become more spiritual and meditate daily.

Transformation and Pearls of Wisdom

Do your best to manage fear, calm down. You don't have to make a decision today. Don't let your fear drive the decision-making process. Interview a lot of doctors. Get numerous and different opinions. Pick a lead doctor, be clear and get various perspectives.

Patrick closed Hollie's interview by saying: "There is deep science behind the treatments we did and there are plenty of studies that support herbal remedies. You can't do a Phase 3 study of all the different things Hollie did. She is an individual and a study of one, but there are many studies of one."

CHRIS

Chris Wark
Colon Cancer
Diagnosed in 2003

"There are no alternatives.
If you don't do chemotherapy, you are insane."
~Doctor's opinion

His Early Years Chris grew up in Germantown, Tennessee, near Memphis. He was an only child, and had a relatively stable, normal upbringing. He attended the University of Tennessee, then the University of Memphis. Upon graduation in 2001, he married at the age of 24, went into the real estate business and started buying properties, fixing them up and selling them. Life was good. Chris was happily married, making his way in the real estate world, without woes or cares. He was living the American dream in Tennessee with nothing but a happy, bright future ahead.

Warning Signs On December 3rd, 2003, Chris started having occasional, deep abdominal pain. The pain was not always present; therefore he delayed investigating its cause, hoping it would eventually go away. Sometimes it was mild discomfort, then a momentary sharp pain. He lived with the intermittent pain for about six months. As the pain escalated, in late December of 2003, his wife convinced him to see a doctor. The first doctor could not identify any reason for the escalating discomfort. Then, Chris made an appointment with a gastroenterologist who performed a colonoscopy and an endoscopy.

Meet Chris

The tests indicated I had a golf ball size tumor in my large intestine, and descending colon. I had a biopsy that confirmed my worst fears. The news was shocking. I was only 26 years old.

The doctor called two days later and said, "You have cancer. Get it removed. I will refer you to a surgeon." My dad also knew a surgeon. I went with my dad's recommendation, and scheduled surgery for New Year's Eve. I had the surgery, and was faced with even worse news: The cancer had spread to my lymph nodes.

I had not eaten in a few days. The first meal the hospital served me was a sloppy joe. I could not believe it, I had just had my intestines sliced and diced and they serve me this sloppy joe.

To Do or Not to Do Chemo: That is the Question

Soon after surgery, I made an appointment with an oncologist. The oncologist said, "You need to do chemo." Prior to his statement, I was thinking that maybe I didn't want to do chemo. My perspective was that it poisons you and your hair falls out. I knew it was very toxic. My feeling was that you can't poison your way to health.

A few days after surgery, my wife and I sat down on the couch, praying and hoping God would open the door to other treatments besides chemotherapy. A couple of days later, a book arrived on my front doorstep from a man who lives in Alaska; a man whom I had never met. A man who knew my father told this man from Alaska about my situation. The book, authored by a health crusader, was about natural therapies and raw vegan diets. It was called *God's Way to Ultimate Health*.

I just broke down on the couch. I felt this book with its message was an answer to my prayer. I called my wife and said, "I am not going to do chemo. I have found a different approach."

Family Pressure

My wife was not happy with my decision. Neither were my family and friends. They said, "Alternative therapies don't work. You must do chemo."

Tremendous psychological and emotional pressure, almost like an intervention, is what I faced from family and friends.

In the face of adverse opinions, I did not want to sound or look like a fool. This was a very difficult time for me. As a compromise with my family, I agreed to an appointment with another oncologist. He had a very nice waiting room, and I noticed everyone in the room was older than me.

As I sat there with my wife, the noisy television in the corner was on "The Today Show." Jack LaLanne came on and started talking about the fact that we are sick is because of the food we eat and that we need to drink lots of freshly made juice, eat raw fresh vegetables and whole fruit to regain our health.

My turn came; the receptionist called my name and I went in to see the oncologist. I asked him about alternatives to chemo. He said, "There are no alternatives. If you don't do chemotherapy you are insane." He was using fear to get me to take action, and he was using the fear of death to get me to sign on with the chemo program.

My wife asked about a raw food diet. He said, "A raw food diet will fight the chemo," meaning, stay away from it, because it will nullify the benefits of the chemo. He proceeded to say, "I am not telling you this because I need your business."

His comments disturbed me. Nonetheless, I was frightened and set up an appointment for a couple weeks later, to put in a port to start the chemo treatments.

Then I went out to the car, sat in the front seat and cried with my wife. I was full of fear and doubt.

Within a week I threw out all the junk food in the house. I started juicing 64 ounces per day, mostly carrots and other veggies. I had huge salads for lunch and dinner to build up my body. I canceled the appointment to put in the port and then had a follow-up appointment with my surgeon. He also tried to use fear to get me to go down the chemo road. He implied, if I did not do this, I would die.

I was always a bit of a non-conformist; I was kicked out of a private school. I did not fit the mold. I was not a follower, and I questioned the status quo frequently. I was into art and music, different from most of the other kids who made fun of me.

Supportive Mom

No one supported my path except my mom. She was always into health products. My mom is an information junkie, a big supporter of natural therapies. That has been her way. My wife had no knowledge of these things and was not supportive of my decisions. She would have preferred, at that time, that I take the conventional path.

Everyone was telling me I was crazy except my mom.

Natural Approach and Changes

I was happy to find a medical professional who agreed with my path. He was and is a great ally. I started seeing him every two weeks. He evaluated my blood, stool and hair, and looked at my entire body. He recommended different supplements, including herbal supplements to detox the liver and other organs, and to strengthen my body. I took aloe vera juice, copious amounts of green powders, chlorella, wheat grass every day, Primal Defense probiotics, mushroom extracts, immune boosting and detox supplements, garlic, cayenne pepper, vitamin D3, vitamin C and other supplements.

Chris's mother suggested, in February of 2004, that Chris should go see a naturopathic doctor and master herbalist in the Memphis area named John Smothers, CTN, M.H. It turned out to be a great recommendation.

For the first 90 days, Dr. Smothers suggested that I follow a 100 percent raw vegan diet. After that, I had some clean, organic meats like free range, organic chicken and lamb. Since that time, I have eaten an 80 percent raw vegan and 20 percent clean meats diet. I also drink lots of veggie drinks (mostly vegetables and sometimes carrots), lots of green tea, red tea, and Jason Winters tea.

> Dr. Smothers proved to be a cornucopia of information for Chris. He also recommended an integrative oncologist, Roy Page, M.D., who suggested a variety of complementary therapies such as: Chinese medicine, vitamin C, IV treatments, specific phytonutrients and other alternatives. Every month Dr. Page monitored Chris's blood to assess his progress. In just a few months, Chris's white blood cell counts improved, markedly.

I was hard-core with my diet, even at family gatherings. I would only eat "my food." My family was kind of silent on the issue. They were glad I attended gatherings, but did not discuss my alternative approach. They let up after a few months and behind my back would say, "He is stubborn and hard-headed. He will just do what he is going to do."

> Family and friends asked Chris early on and repeatedly: "Why don't you want to do chemotherapy?" His response: "Because I want to live."

People don't realize that chemotherapy and radiation are destructive to the body. They are cancer-causing treatments. They may bring about No Evidence of Disease (NED) within a few months or years, but frequently the cancer comes back with a vengeance, harsher than ever.

I did rebounding (which is a low-impact exercise on a mini-trampoline) every day, two to three times per day. It moves the lymphatic system. I also ran one mile every morning and went to a sauna several days per week to sweat out toxins. I threw out my conventional toothpaste and shampoo. I cleaned up the water, reduced all toxic exposure in the house and cleaned up my environment to limit exposure to external toxins.

I still take a ton of supplements. I rotate different supplements in and out. Now, I take curcumin, quercetin, Poly MVA, selenium, liposomal vitamin C, raw whole food, multivitamins, flax seed in my smoothies, moringa and assorted other things. I still have blood work once per year. After Dr. Page died, I decided to see another oncologist, Donald Gravenor, M.D., a conventional yet open-minded doctor. I still see Dr. Smothers every few months.

Transformation and Pearls of Wisdom

This experience has made me realize how critical food is to your health. I spend a lot of time blogging about health, sharing my story and getting information to people so they can make major lifestyle changes, before they get into trouble.

> The cancer tribulations and evolutionary path Chris has traveled changed him—dramatically. He has become a well-known advocate for integrative and alternative cancer therapies. He speaks at national cancer conferences, has made appearances on television talk shows, and posts his opinions and articles frequently to his active blog. He has two young, beautiful daughters and an adoring wife.

We live in a very toxic world. Toxins exist in our foods and in the products we use everyday. Most of the food we eat has zero nutrients. Feed your body real organic fruits and vegetables, clean meats and clean water. Reduce the exposure in your home to the unhealthy products we use. Eliminate toxic relationships and toxic emotions, including resentment, guilt, envy and bitterness. When you harbor these emotions, they will ultimately bring about poor health.

You need to make good choices every day.
It is not easy; it is the tougher road.

Fast food is too easy; stay on top of good healthy choices. Going through this has changed my attitude about life. I am happy to be alive. I don't need a big house; it is not that important to me. The best way to make yourself miserable is to focus on things you can't have or that you want.

Count your blessings and take stock of all the good things you have in your life; then the trivial frustrating events of the day won't matter.

JANET

Janet Vitt Sommer
Metastatic Lung Cancer
Diagnosed in 1995

"You have three to six weeks to live."
~Doctor's prognosis at a major cancer hospital in the Midwest

Her Early Years Born in 1950, Janet Vitt grew up near Cleveland, Ohio with her brother and sister. The family was raised Catholic. She and her siblings attended religious school and church on a regular basis.

Janet's parents smoked three packs of cigarettes every day. Although Janet was never a smoker, she recalls breathing lots of secondary smoke during her early years. She was also exposed to secondary smoke during her tenure as a nurse between 1971 and 1995; many nurses she worked with were habitual smokers.

Janet had a poor diet, eating lots of dairy and excessive amounts of cheese. She always assumed she was healthy because she never smoked cigarettes and was always slender. Breakfast generally consisted solely of coffee. She ate lunch sporadically and would try to find time to eat dinner, usually late at night.

Lifestyle Janet was a nurse manager. She had a full-time job teaching nurses seven days per week how to become "the best nurses possible." She was always on the go, rarely thinking of her own health; she never stopped to smell the flowers. During Janet's late 30s, anxiety and tension were commonplace in her home; she went through a divorce when she reached 40 years of age.

Diagnosis One month before her diagnosis, at the age of 45, Janet felt unusually fatigued. A girlfriend commented, "You know, you clear your throat all the time." The comment caused Janet to think more about her health. She remembered how her lungs felt heavy.

She went to her doctor who initially thought she might have bronchitis. However, after listening to her lungs, which sounded clear, he concluded, "There is no problem."

A recreational tennis player, Janet asked a casual tennis partner (a doctor, but not her doctor) for an antibiotic, because regardless of her doctor's diagnosis that there was no problem, she still felt that she might have bronchitis. He agreed to give her an antibiotic, but strongly suggested she get a CT scan to make sure she did not have pneumonia.

Janet had the CT scan which, shockingly, showed evidence of probable lung cancer. She followed up the CT scan with a PET Scan which brought traumatic news: A mass in her left lung, tumors in both lungs, tumors in her pancreas, stomach, liver and throughout her lymphatic system.

On April 11th, 1995, Janet was diagnosed with lung cancer, non-small cell adenocarcinoma, biopsy-proven and confirmed, again, as a result of the extensive scans.

Meet Janet

I said, "It can't be, I feel OK!" I was absolutely shocked. The doctor said, "You have three to six months to live. There is no hope."

Second Opinion Janet had terminal cancer and could not believe the news. She went for a second opinion at a large cancer center in Cleveland. The news there was even worse. The doctors told her, "You have three to six weeks to live."

I told my two sons that I was going to die. As an experienced practicing nurse and nurse manager, I was not naive about my prospects. I knew they were ominous at best.

On April 18th, 1995, just one week after her diagnosis, Janet had surgery to remove her stomach mass and, shortly thereafter, began chemotherapy even though her doctor said, "It might buy only a month or two."

Chemo Side Effects The plan was to engage in six treatments of chemo, Taxol and carboplatin. She was given one dose, but within three weeks, Janet lost over 35 percent of her body weight, going from 114 to 72 pounds. She was incredibly frail at 72 pounds and 5'6" tall.

I looked like a concentration camp survivor. It was impossible for me to continue the chemotherapy treatments.

Hospice Care Before leaving the hospital, she agreed to enter hospice care. The hospice nurses and practitioners were angels. They put together a schedule for Janet and came to her house daily. She was given "no chance" to live more than a very short time.

Alternative Therapy

Despite my hopeless prognosis, my doctor, Dennis Grossman, M.D. said, "Why don't you try something alternative?"

I said, "I can't do that [alternative treatment]. That is for hippies." I was trained conventionally and taught that anything besides allopathic medicine was mere nonsense.

My doctor said, "You have nothing to lose. Why don't you look into macrobiotic food?" Reluctantly, but with encouragement from my sister Nancy, who was in the room when the recommendation was made, I sought out a macrobiotic counselor from the phone book.

In her weakened state, Janet listened to the counselor with skepticism. Regardless, Francois Roland, from the Cleveland area, was able to inform and educate Janet about the benefits of a macrobiotic diet.

He gave me and my friends cooking classes. He did not promise a miracle cure, but he gave me hope. I will never forget the words he said to me: "You can be healed."

I was very weak, my lungs were filled with fluid, I had difficulty breathing, I was on oxygen, using a wheelchair, a shower chair and needed help to get to the bathroom.

I was very lucky to have an incredible support system of eight different friends who watched over me on a scheduled basis every day. My friends cooked for me and did not deviate from the diet one bit.

Essentially, the diet excluded dairy, meat, sugar and other foods. It included whole grains, beans, organic fresh vegetables and other specific healing foods. Janet's sister eliminated everything related to the "standard America diet" from her home.

Remarkably, two days after I started on the diet I stopped my constant vomiting; in fact, I stopped altogether! Suddenly I felt better and decided, in a moment of clarity, 10 days into the diet, to flush all of my drugs down the toilet. The anti-anxiety drugs, the pain medication, the diuretic drugs and many others. I felt, "This is my only shot," and I didn't want to stress my liver with these drugs. I still had pain, but felt better and decided, "I can't be mean to my liver." I was extremely weak, but stayed with the diet.

I instructed my loved ones not to resuscitate me and not to call 9-1-1 if I stopped breathing.

During the first five months on the diet my tumors kept growing, but slowly. I kept getting hospice care and stayed with the diet. At this point, I did not want any more bad news, so I instructed my doctor that I did not want any more scans.

I was now into deep breathing and prayer. I also had frequent full body massages, which were soothing. Deep breathing helped alleviate my pain and helped me relax. Prior to this experience, as a skeptic, and as a conventional practicing nurse, I never believed deep breathing could be helpful.

"All Your Tumors are Gone!"

Time marched on. I was still very weak, but my friends cooked healthy macrobiotic meals, every meal, seven days a week. Ten months had now elapsed since I began the diet and one year had elapsed since my diagnosis. I decided to get scanned to see what was going on. I was scared, but also curious; after all, I had lived longer than most expected. A few days later, at 9:30 in the evening, my doctor called and gave me startling news:

"All your tumors are gone!" Those were the best words I heard in my life besides, 'It's a boy!'"

I couldn't believe it. I now felt there is validity to this diet. I now wanted to know, "Why does this work?" Before I was told, "Your tumors are gone," I didn't really care. I just wanted some palliative relief.

During my first year in hospice, I gave away many clothes, thinking I was a goner. I learned that "stuff" is not important. I became more trusting with people. I was very fortunate that I had a great support group, eight people, including my sister, who would cook for me, do my laundry and other tedious chores in the 12 months since my diagnosis. I was in hospice care for 18 months. Eighteen months! After completing hospice care, I started walking every day; I had been too weak until that point.

Tumor Board Presentation

My internist asked if I wanted to present my case to the tumor board at University Bedford Hospital in Cleveland. The board included approximately 15 people, including doctors, nurses, oncologists, hospice workers and others. I said, "Yes!" My doctor (the internist) presented my case from his viewpoint and I did so from mine.

The initial scans and then the clean scans were shown at the presentation. One doctor said, "It is impossible that this is the same person." Fractures in the ribs were visible from both scans, substantiating the validity of the scans. I had fractured my ribs many years before and this was a factor in convincing the board that yes, this was me.

Another doctor rationalized, "It must have been the one dose of chemo that did the trick." Another doctor said, "That doesn't make sense, because when we give all six treatments for this type of metastasized cancer, six cycles don't work anyway."

One doctor said, "It was caused by spontaneous healing." That is code for, "We don't know why she healed and it is unexplainable from a conventional viewpoint."

My doctor said, "Whatever the cause, she is here and this is what she did."

Transformation and Pearls of Wisdom

It has now been 21 years since my diagnosis, and I will never go off the diet. I have friends who were on the diet, and their tumors disappeared. Then, they went off of the diet and the tumors came back. They died.

In May 1996, I went to the Kushi Institute in Massachusetts (the leading macrobiotic educational center in the world) and took classes. It was great to be with people who were new to this. I loved learning everything about the diet, the reasons why it works and telling my story to people new to the diet who had a sincere interest in learning.

I truly believe how I eat impacts every cell in my body. I am now more open and trusting. I used to be cynical, skeptical and an angry person. I believe anything is possible. I thank God for my story, because it gives people hope.

I never would have tried integrative or alternative therapies, but my doctor suggested it.

I thank God my doctor was open-minded and encouraged me to explore macrobiotics. I believe there is more than one way to heal cancer. When you feel comfortable about a path, go with it, or several paths. I believe nutrition is something we all have in common; it makes a huge difference in your life. Unfortunately we eat like pigs in America. We eat on the run, we eat standing up, we overeat and "supersize" ourselves.

Since I left hospice, life has been great. People who embrace this lifestyle heal! But, they must stay with it 100 percent. The key word is "embrace." They must embrace the program. I have witnessed so much as a macrobiotic teacher and counselor. It is a gift to me to see people heal from cancer, heart disease, MS, and diabetes.

When people clean up their acts, people heal. Now, I go on frequent bike rides with my new husband. His former wife died of cancer. When I met him he weighed 200 pounds and had a 36-inch waist. I got him on the diet and he is now 160 pounds and has a 30-inch waist!

I thank God every morning for the new day, before my feet hit the floor. It puts gratitude in my heart.

At the end of our interview, Janet said, "Never give up. Never ever give up!"

ANN

Ann Fonfa
Breast Cancer
Diagnosed in 1993

"If you don't do chemo, you will die."
"If you don't do radiation, you will die."
~Two different doctors of Ann's in NYC

Her Early Years Ann was born in Queens and grew up in New York City. She is the oldest of three children. Heart disease was prevalent in her family; not cancer.

Meet Ann

My definition of a healthy vegetable eater was quite different when I was in my twenties. I thought adding iceberg lettuce, tomato, mayonnaise, and rye bread to a cheeseburger made me a healthy eater.

Cancer Discovered

In 1989, I discovered I had a serious chemical sensitivity. To this day I have problems being around people who use deodorant, perfume, cologne and other products with chemicals. Exposure would often make me sick; I would have to stay in bed for many days at a time.

My perception in the 1990s was that you couldn't get cancer unless your mother had it. I was quite naive and knew nothing about it. I also knew nothing about alternative treatments or therapies.

In 1991, I went to an acupuncturist who was also a friend of mine. She took away my menstrual cramps of 30 years; I was quite impressed.

In late December of 1992, I felt something funny in my breast. A few weeks later, on January 11th, 1993, I went to get a mammogram. I was only 44 years old. After the mammogram, my doctor pushed me to see a breast surgeon who recommended a lumpectomy. He said, "You may have cancer." This was very surprising.

Surgery
Surgery was scheduled for 10:00 a.m. at the Beth Israel Hospital in New York City. The surgeon removed the cancerous lump and 18 lymph nodes that were negative. I was told I had Stage 1 invasive lobular carcinoma.

As a result of the doctor's removing so many lymph nodes, I developed and still suffer from lymphedema. Lymphedema is a permanent swelling of the arm (although lymphedema can occur in other parts of the body, too). My left arm is swollen and not as strong as my right arm. I suffer from pain and discomfort from time to time. It is difficult to carry things and by the end of the day, it can be quite difficult to lift my arm.

Do Chemotherapy and/or Radiation or "You will die"
Shortly after surgery, I saw an oncologist. He wanted me to start chemo right away. I said, "No, I have chemical sensitivity to many things and I don't want to do chemotherapy." He said my chemical sensitivity was irrelevant, that it didn't matter. This doctor said, "If you don't do chemotherapy, you will die." I was not persuaded.

Shortly thereafter, in February of 1993, I went to a cancer support group. I told the people in the group that I refused chemo and they said, "You must do something."

I contemplated radiation. I went to the radiation wing at Beth Israel where you are measured for radiation. There was an old machine and a new machine. The person who was measuring patients was a student, not an expert. This made me very nervous.

Later, on a drive up to Boston, I decided not to do radiation, especially since I learned that my heart would be in the radiation field. Also, I had read a report issued by the National Surgical Adjuvant Breast and Bowel Project that described the results of an 8-year study comparing getting a mastectomy, or lumpectomy with and without radiation. At that time, the overall survival for each was the same.

As a result, I did not go down the radiation road and did not get a mastectomy either, at that time. My doctor was so upset. He called my husband, Steve, and told him, "Your wife will die if she does not do radiation." I decided I must find other alternatives, but not chemotherapy or radiation.

Taking Control, Being Proactive, and Learning In 1994, just over a year since diagnosis, Ann became more proactive and mindful about her health and her lifestyle.

I started eating only organic foods, and rarely sweets. No meat, chicken or turkey. Occasional fish, but no dairy. In 1995, I decided to take detoxification very seriously. Detox is critical. I have engaged in taking coffee enemas for detox since 1995.

I started a support group. I advertised its existence in a self-help support newsletter, *SHARE*. Seventy women showed up at the first meeting. I brought in many different speakers, including acupuncturists, practitioners from Mexican clinics, herbalists, other practitioners and other alternative advocates.

I then founded an organization called the "Annie Appleseed Project." I put together a 63-page summary of natural therapies and made 100 copies to hand out to people. I am a talker and like to share information with people. This was the real beginning of my organization.

In 1995, I also had a local recurrence, the first of a series of local tumor recurrences in the breast and chest wall area. I attempted to control the recurrences with metabolic enzyme therapy and then 714X treatments in Canada, but they didn't work. The biopsy-proven tumors continued to grow, albeit slowly.

After two more lumpectomies, I decided to have a mastectomy. Approximately 10 months later, the other breast developed Paget's disease of the nipple. This usually indicates a malignant tumor, but none was found.

In 1993, Ann was diagnosed with Stage 1 breast cancer. In 1997, she was diagnosed with Stage 4 breast cancer. She was now faced with a daunting challenge; a most serious nerve-wracking reality.

A few months later, Ann began treatment with the Gerson Clinic in Mexico, a well-known clinic founded upon the principles of Max Gerson, M.D. who began treating cancer patients around 1928. His daughter, Charlotte, founded the Gerson Institute in 1977.

Gerson Clinic

I spent two weeks at Gerson, accompanied by my mother. The treatments consisted of a highly specified organic meal plan, injections, supplements, lots of juicing throughout the day, hydrotherapy, lectures, check-ups with doctors, coffee enemas, Coley's Toxins, IV vitamin C, and other things, depending upon the patient's cancer and condition. Many of the people at the clinic were very sick, many with mets (metastasized cancer). The people at the clinic were very warm and loving, truly sincere and caring.

Back in New York, I continued to juice 13 times per day, gave myself shots, ate a very clean diet, and gave myself enemas every day. It is a very tough 18-month regimen.

Profits Over Patients

Unless they can patent a drug, pharmaceutical companies will not give credit to any treatment or product which may be beneficial to cancer patients. Is it about us or is it about making money? It is important to ask questions; to make sure you are getting the truth.

I have been at meetings where pharmaceutical representatives have said to me, "We can't patent that treatment or supplement or natural therapy, so we are not going to endorse it."

There is no magic bullet. People can die from anything, but it will be a combination of things that make you healthy.

The Paradox of Perception

When people die of cancer who were treated conventionally, the obituary says, "They fought a valiant fight." When people die of cancer who were treated alternatively, the common judgment is, "They did alternative and died; alternative was worthless." Of course, this is after they were told by their doctor they would die, because their cancer had metastasized and became terminal.

The great majority of people who die every year from cancer, die despite implementing conventional treatments, because most people only follow a conventional path.

Cancer death rates are not properly reported. Many people die of complications related to cancer. Also, sometimes, the actual conventional cancer treatments cause cancer.

Dr. George Wong, Traditional Chinese Medicine

I first met George Wong, Ph.D. at the San Antonio Breast Cancer Conference in 1998. After telling him about my medical history, he asked me to work with him. His family was deeply associated with the medical field, including M.D.s, Ph.D.s, and herbalists.

I hesitated, although I was impressed with the fact that he had a a Master's and Ph.D. from Harvard University, was a Professor with the Weill Cornell Medical College, had worked previously at Memorial Sloan Kettering Cancer Center and had other noteworthy accomplishments. Additionally, he was a fourth generation Chinese herbalist.

At that time, I was suffering from recurrent, and what had been called Stage 4 breast cancer, due to chest wall tumors. He told me that he thought he could help me and would like to try. I was aware of the value of acupuncture, but had no idea about Chinese herbs.

By April 1999, I felt "enough was enough." I had just developed my 25th tumor. I called Dr. Wong, but first I had an MRI to show where the cancer currently was; the scan confirmed a 3.5 cm "area of involvement."

Dr. Wong met with me and ended up giving me an herbal prescription. I made the herbal tea and after drinking it, got hives all over my body. I was very frightened by this, but within three days it was obvious that I had received a health benefit. My very severe multiple chemical sensitivities and symptoms had changed, and the intensity of the symptoms was reduced by approximately 60 percent.

No longer would I have to crawl into bed for days, nauseated and with serious headaches after smelling something that troubled me. I now only had mild headaches that went away in moments, rather than days. I started taking the herbs again, not willing to stop even when Dr. Wong suggested I could.

The Irony of 9/11

I had an appointment with my doctor on 9/12/01, one day after 9/11. On 9/12, I was told, "You are cancer free, no discernible evidence of disease."

I started to cry. People thought I was crying because of the horrific events of 9/11, but I was crying about being told I was cancer free after experiencing five years of recurrences, over and over. Now they could not see any cancer in my body. I was so relieved.

> **There is so much evidence about the value of exercise, healthy food, mind-body efforts, detoxification, supplements, vitamins and other things that can help fight cancer. There is so much you can do to help yourself.**

Transformation and Pearls of Wisdom

Change what you eat. Add more fruits and vegetables, be physically active every day, find ways to relax; everyone needs to focus on being well and staying with a program. Make the commitment to yourself and stay with it. Live every day. You must be eternally vigilant and stay with the program. You can't go backwards and eat junk. Throw away all the bad food in your house and all of the toxic products.

According to the American Cancer Society, only 12 percent of the population eats the recommended five to nine vegetables and fruits per day we should eat.

We were not meant to eat donuts!

Everyone should take fish oil, probiotics, and curcumin, as well as acupuncture. Lots of studies show vitamins, nutrients, and supplements are very helpful. You can't be afraid to take these helpful supplements.

Make sure you ask doctors, "What are the expectations from taking the conventional treatments?" The cancer mortality rate is very high. There has been virtually no change in years, yet we continue with chemo and radiation, knowing that for many the survival benefit is minimal.

There is a necessity for people to learn about complementary and alternative treatments. There are many paths to wellness.

BARB

Barb Pytlewski
**Multiple Cancers: Uterine, Colon and Ureters, with Metastases
to the Lungs, Pelvis, Kidney and Liver**
Diagnosed in 1988

"You have about two years to live."
~Doctor's prognosis at a major cancer center

Her Early Years Barb is the middle child of three siblings. She was born in Newark, New Jersey to a first generation American-Italian father and first generation American-Yugoslavian mother. Her father was an engineer and her mother a "beautiful, gutsy gal," according to Barb. The family was quite musical, always listening to classical music.

During her early years, Barb had very serious asthma issues. She almost died several times between ages 2 and 7, but she says, "by the grace of God, I had the will to live, which I received from my gutsy mom."

When Barb turned 12, the family moved to Southern California, a better climate for her troubling asthma condition.

Meet Barb

When we moved to Los Angeles, my dad went to work for Rockwell. I was into music and ultimately received a degree from the University of Southern California in performance. I played the bassoon and was involved in live performances. Later in life, I also took up the harp. My sister was a concert pianist and my brother became a computer tech.

During the course of my life, I have had the honor of playing music at the Aspen Music Festival in the chamber symphony. I have also played in the Sun Valley Symphony, and with orchestras in Los Angeles, Utah, and Las Vegas as well as with other notable musical groups.

On a different note, I also got my hands dirty and drove a tractor at my first husband's and my ranch near Bozeman, Montana. I have always been involved in many interesting activities my whole life.

As a child, I was exposed to cancer throughout the family. My grandmother died from a gynecological cancer. Two aunts died of cancer. An uncle died of cancer and eight cousins also died of cancer. When my brother was 22 years old, he was diagnosed with testicular cancer; fortunately he survived. The word "cancer" has always struck fear in my heart.

> At the age of 42, Barb was living in Sun Valley, Idaho. She and her husband had two adopted daughters—7 years old and 9 months old.

Diagnosis: Stage 1 Uterine Cancer

My marriage was in good shape, I was exercising and eating relatively healthy food, but I was bleeding between my periods. I was concerned.

Her doctors were concerned with the initial test results and decided to examine Barb more closely. She had a biopsy and was diagnosed with Stage 1 uterine cancer.

> Previously, Barb's brother had been successfully treated for testicular cancer at UCLA. Since Barb had graduated from USC, just a few miles from UCLA, she felt comfortable with the medical treatments she might receive in Los Angeles. Despite the fact she was living in Idaho at the time, she decided to travel to Los Angeles for treatment.

My treatment entailed a radical hysterectomy at St. Joseph's Hospital in Burbank. It was a horrific surgery.

Temporary Respite, Then Fears are Realized

Time marched on. Everything was fine for 15 years. Then, my brother was diagnosed with colon cancer in 2003. I was getting quite nervous about a familial connection with cancers related to the digestive system. I had been having colonoscopies every few years due to my family's history.

In the fall of 2008, I was due for a colonoscopy. I had been feeling a bit lethargic and sleepy. I went to my husband's internist for a physical and blood work. He called me a few days later and said there was something wrong; the test results were abnormal. I had the colonoscopy and a tumor was found. I had colon cancer.

My gastroenterologist in Salt Lake City said to me, "I know you have microsatellite instability." It also means I may have Lynch Syndrome, an inherited condition that increases one's risk of colon and other cancers. The doctor recommended removal of my entire colon. I said no. Instead of a radical procedure to remove my entire colon, I had a right colectomy: the removal or excision of part of my colon. When performing the colectomy, the surgeons noticed that both of my ureters looked strange; kind of lumpy. They performed a biopsy of the ureters and reported no cancer, but another doctor said, "It must be cancerous."

In the meantime, the urologist put in stents to keep the ureters open. At this time, we were living in Las Vegas and my husband lost his job in architecture due to the recession. It was a very stressful time.

Problems never ceased for Barb. On December 3rd, 2008 she had exploratory surgery in Salt Lake City. The urologic surgery confirmed she had bilateral cancer of the ureters, contrary to the earlier surgeon who stated that she did not have cancer of the ureters. Now, to complicate matters, Barb had the distinction of four cancers in her medical records: uterine cancer, colon cancer, including left and right ureter cancer, very rare and deadly.

More Cancer and a Death Sentence

Now, I was given a death sentence. A doctor in Salt Lake said, "You have about two years to live." He recommended a chemotherapy treatment that might bring about the direct effect of destroying whatever kidney function I had remaining.

Cancer had already destroyed my left kidney. Then he recommended taking out the entire urinary system and having me go on dialysis. He also wanted to give me Cisplatin. He held virtually no hope for me.

A Rare Surgical Procedure at UCLA and Again, Yes, More Cancers

First, I called the University of Utah to try and see an expert, but they couldn't see me for a month. I wasn't going to wait a month. Time was too precious. I headed back to Los Angeles, specifically to see the doctors at the Clark Urology Center at UCLA, hoping they might be able to help me.

I was not about to give up.

I called and got the receptionist on the phone. I explained that I had bilateral cancer of the ureters. She was an angel who arranged an appointment with a famous urologic surgeon who had saved many lives.

He is an extremely rare man, a genius, a humanitarian. He asked me, "What do you want?," I said, "At least five years."

I went to the Rose Bowl Parade on January 1st, 2009 and had major surgery on January 5th. When I came out of surgery I was in kidney failure, near death, in excruciating pain, with all kinds of lines and intravenous tubes coming out of my body. I was in the hospital for almost a month, and just one day from going on dialysis. The doctors wondered if I would die in the hospital.

I turned the corner and my right kidney started to work, but I contracted C. difficile (Clostridium difficile, or C. diff, a very serious infectious diarrhea). I was quarantined. It was horrendous.

Only three months before, I had colon cancer and now a long segment of my small intestine was removed to fashion replacement ureters. The cancer extended up going into the renal pelvis area of both kidneys. This presented a very grave situation for me. I lost a tremendous amount of weight. Although the kidney started to work, I had Stage 3 cancer in my left ureter and Stage 2 cancer in the right ureter. My bladder had to be restructured. My surgeon said there are very few people in the United States "walking around with plumbing like you."

At that time, there had only been 50 surgeries in the country where both ureters (bilateral replacement) had taken place at the same time. Fortunately, my wonderful urologic surgeon had handled approximately 15 of them.

I also had bladder tumors that had to be removed during the ureter surgery. Once you have had ureter cancer, the area is fertile ground for more tumors. My bladder did not empty on its own once the kidney started working. For two months I had to self-catheterize. Finally, over time, the bladder began to work again.

I went home to a retirement home in Colorado and started to get back to life in Glenwood Springs. You can't expect your doctor to play God and do everything for you. You must be proactive and have an insatiable desire to find out and do everything you can for yourself.

When I got the pathology report in March, 2009, the CT scan showed that I might have had metastases to the liver and lungs. When I asked the surgeon why he hadn't sent me to the oncologist for chemo, he said, "Because you would have died." He said the prognosis was not good before surgery and he did not believe I would live very long.

In June, 2009, when I went back for another CT scan, unfortunately lesions were strongly suspected on the liver, with some confirmed in the lungs, pelvis and left kidney. Next, I was sent to an oncologist at UCLA. He told me, "You probably have two years to live."

Barb was in a most improbable quandary. She lived in an impenetrable fog, on an emotional rollercoaster, and in excruciating pain. She continuously traveled in a medically uncertain direction. She had multiple types of serious cancer, was given a two-year death sentence in December 2008 and again in June 2009 by different doctors. She had also suffered through a rare and most challenging surgery. To say the future looked bleak was a gross understatement.

Complementary Recommendations from Dr. Jeanne Wallace

In June of 2008, I was reading a book review in the *Los Angeles Times* titled "AntiCancer: A New Way of Life," by David Servan-Schreiber, M.D. At the back of the actual book, in the Acknowledgments, he thanked Jeanne Wallace, Ph.D. for her impressive work and how it had changed his life.

I immediately went on the Internet to find her, and talked to her before my surgery. She encouraged me to call her after my surgery.

When I was told I had two years to live with metastatic disease in June 2009, I decided to call Jeanne Wallace again. I told her I was starting chemo soon, and I needed her help. I sent her all kinds of notes about my diagnosis, type of tumor, stage and other related information. She wanted to know the exact protocol being prescribed.

I could not do Cisplatin due to my kidney problems. There was a 10 percent survival record for Cisplatin, with Stage 4 metastatic disease, but no record of survival for Carboplatin and Gemzar which was the chemo cocktail of choice.

After one round the doctors stopped, I had to get Neupogin shots to build white cells quicker. After two cycles of chemo I contracted salmonella. In December of 2009, my oncologist at the Los Angeles Clinic, affiliated with Santa Monica Hospital, said, "We can't give you any more."

Jeanne Wallace recommended many evidence-based supplements and vitamins to boost my cells, and to protect my bone marrow. She also made recommendations to protect my right kidney, to mitigate nausea and constipation.

One recommendation, among others, to help with nausea and boost my immune system, was acupuncture. She also helped me prevent nerve damage from the chemotherapy and helped keep my internal inflammation down. During the chemo, and ever since, I had and continue to have certain blood tests, recommended by Jeanne to ascertain how I handled the chemo and how my body's internal terrain is handling my disease.

Jeanne has serious peer-reviewed medical reports and literature to support all of her recommendations: real, evidence-based studies to back up her suggestions. Jeanne and her team have helped me so much. She also has given me many excellent, specific recommendations about food and nutrition regarding my cancer and condition.

This is my new diet: no red meat, limited carbs, limited fruit (except I do eat berries), and matcha green tea. I stay away from sugar, I eat almond flour (not other flour), I eat nuts, drink lots of alkaline water and eat lots of veggies, especially cruciferous veggies. I take lots of supplements recommended by Jeanne and her team. Some of the supplements include: vitamin D3, a particular Chinese mushroom herb, resveratrol, selenium, CoQ10, molybdenum, zinc, and other customized supplements.

Of course, everyone's situation is different so it is important to get expert advice about what may be helpful for your personal cancer issues.

During my cancer fight I have consulted with Jeanne's team every two weeks. She educated me about all the things I could do to help balance my body and help my body deal with surgery, chemo, and the cancer.

I learned from her that an integrative approach is best.

If I had never met Jeanne, I would probably not be here today. She and her people are amazing!

In addition to Jeanne's wonderful work, I met Michael Tsuei, also known as Master Tsuei. He is a phenomenal medical qui gong practitioner. In addition to the medical treatments and the other alternative things I do, I exercise a lot. Every day, I do something to try to build up my immune system. I cycle 14 miles per day, six days per week, weather permitting. I also do deep-water aerobics, yoga, cross-country skiing (in the winter), and qi gong stretching whenever possible.

Transformation and Pearls of Wisdom

I appreciate every day of my life. I take nothing for granted. I am a very strong, passionate person. I am very passionate about music and nature. I had pictures of nature in my room at the hospital and listened to music frequently to help me deal with the tremendous pain. I have a high degree of faith. I try to make every day matter. I am aware of breathing in and out without pain, enjoying simple things in life, the blue skies, the trees.

**Life is too important to waste. Life does not go on
forever, so don't worry about silly things.**

Every four months I go to UCLA to get checked out. It can be tedious, but
you must determine if it is worth it or not. It takes hard work. If you don't put
up the fight, you will never know. Many people don't have the will to do it.

I asked Barb what she would recommend to someone who was just
diagnosed with cancer.

She said to find and seek someone like Jeanne. These naturopathic types of
people give you hope. The doctors just give you numbers and statistics. Seek out
things besides traditional medical doctors.

Join a support group. It made a difference to be with people who knew what
I was going through. I had loving support around me. My oncologist said if I
had not been in great shape, my body could not have withstood what I have
been through.

I hold my urologic surgeon, oncologist, Master Tsuei, Dr. Jeanne Wallace
and Michelle Gerencser as the most important people who deserve the credit,
including me, for my survival.

My oncologist now believes the "integrative approach" has had a major impact
on my being here. My surgeon is astounded. He said, "I wish I could clone you,
your attitude and drive. I have rarely seen this in any patient."

You can't expect your doctor to play God and do everything for you. You
must be proactive and have an insatiable desire to find out and do everything
you can for yourself.

**You must be passionate about life to survive. If you
have not adopted a healthy lifestyle, do it. Treat
your body as a temple. Take care of yourself.**

CHERYL

Cheryl Clark
Brain Cancer, Glioblastoma
Diagnosed in 1997

"Get your affairs in order. We can do chemo,
but it is only palliative, short term."
~Doctor in Santa Cruz, California

Her Early Years Cheryl grew up in the Upper Peninsula of Michigan. Her mom was an elementary school teacher and her dad was self-employed. Cheryl was always interested in sports, especially basketball. She played for the University of Southwest Louisiana (now known as the University of Louisiana at Lafayette) where she obtained her college degree with honors.

After college she played professional basketball for a team known as the "All American Redheads Pioneers." She traveled extensively with the team between 1970 until 1982, barnstorming in small venues throughout the United States. In June of 1999, the team was honored as pioneers in women's basketball and inducted into the Women's Basketball Hall of Fame in Nashville, Tennessee.

Additional individual athletic honors were bestowed upon Cheryl; she was also admitted to the UP (Upper Peninsula) Sports Hall of Fame in May of 2001 for her basketball prowess with the All American Redheads Pioneers.

The Incident In October of 1997, Cheryl and her best friend Jeanne Wallace traveled to a beautiful beach resort in Hilton Head, South Carolina to get away from the daily mundane routines of life. While riding horses one sunny afternoon, trekking through the trees next to the beach, Cheryl and Jeanne posed for a photo by the sea. Within one minute, Cheryl was seeing fireworks in her head, as if it were the 4th of July. The 48-year-old athlete was having a seizure; a major seizure.

Meet Cheryl

I fell off my horse, smashing violently onto the beach. I had no pulse, my eyes were wide open, and I was totally unresponsive.

> **I saw bright white lights. I saw my parents walking over to me and my mother said, 'No, no, not now, go back, go back.' I was immersed in a near death experience.**

All of a sudden, I recovered consciousness. I had broken my spine at the 8th vertebra, fractured eight ribs and my spine almost snapped; it was hanging on by a thread. I was rushed to Savannah, Georgia, about 45 minutes away. My situation was too critical for any hospital in Hilton Head.

I was scanned up and down my body that night. The really bad news was about to be uncovered. The doctors discovered a large hemorrhaging, lemon-sized tumor in my brain. I was in the ICU at Memorial Medical Center for five days. My breathing was shallow and the doctors had to constantly drain blood from my lungs.

After those five days, I had brain surgery in Savannah. The location of the brain tumor was above the right ear in the right temporal lobe. During my surgery, I had a dream or hallucination. Jesus appeared and said, "You will be OK." At that moment, I had no doubt I would survive long term.

In addition to my brain surgery, I also underwent major back surgery and had my vertebrae fused together. Post surgery, the pathology report came back indicating a devastating diagnosis: Glioblastoma Multiforme (GBM IV), the worst and most aggressive kind of malignant brain tumor. I had grade 4 brain cancer.

My prognosis?

I was told I had six to nine months to live. I had no warning, and now, I was staring into the abyss with no way out. I was only 48 years old.

Get Your Affairs in Order

I was living in California at the time and when I was able to get out of the hospital in Savannah, I was referred to an oncologist in Santa Cruz. This doctor's prognosis was grave at best. He told me, "Get your affairs in order." He said, "We can do chemo, but it is only palliative, short term. Nothing serious can be done." He was very negative about any treatment or therapy that might be helpful.

I was angry and very upset. I would not accept this as fact. I fired him. I needed someone who felt there might be a path to survival. My health was not good. I lost 30 pounds from the time I fell off the horse until my meeting with my oncologist in Santa Cruz. I went from 161 to 131 pounds.

Protocol: Making Choices

These were trying times, with great uncertainty and adversity, but Cheryl was steely and unyielding in her determination to find a hopeful path as she faced this most daunting foe.

A respected oncologist gave me no hope and everyone knows GBMs are viewed as death sentences. Still, I would not give up.

I was determined and very fortunate to have a great ally in my best friend, Jeanne Wallace, since she was, and is, an expert in educating people about the great benefits of nutritional science, especially concerning cancer, her specialty. I worked closely with Jeanne in all of my decisions.

I chose not to do chemo because I felt it would do more harm than good. Instead, I chose to engage in a radiation protocol despite the conventional consensus that it, too, was not considered anything more than palliative. However, I gave it a shot, combined with lots of other complementary therapies. My radiation oncologist was against supplementation of any kind during my radiation treatments, but Jeanne and I ultimately persuaded him to permit Jeanne to implement her nutritional and supplementation program for me despite his reluctance.

I waited six months before undergoing radiation, even though my former oncologist said I would be dead in six to nine months. I wanted to do everything possible prior to radiation to boost my immune system.

Right after my seizure, I began working on transforming my health. As soon as I left the hospital in Savannah, I began a serious supplementation program developed by Jeanne. I went through radiation and did not have any significant side effects due to the protective nutritional actions taken prior to my treatments.

Jeanne deserves great credit for her nutritional recommendations and scientifically based supplementation protocol. After my traditional radiation, we (Jeanne and I) heard about a clinical trial conducted in 1997, using gamma knife radiation therapy. I engaged in this one, as well.

The treatments and therapies that became part of my regimen—before, during and after my radiation—were not randomly chosen. They were all selected and designed to do different things, including: slow tumor growth, strengthen my immune system, inhibit angiogenesis, slow and eliminate out-of-control inflammation, enhance cell differentiation, promote apoptosis, protect healthy brain tissue from radiation, enhance oxygen rich blood to my system, promote a positive attitude, and other direct and indirect medicinal benefits.

Mind-body exercises were and are also very important for me.

When the mind gives up, the body follows. This relationship is critical. Calm your fears. I decided to fill my mind with positive thoughts.

I frequently engaged in visualizations, affirmations, laughter, and the reading of dozens of survivor success stories. You can choose to be up or you can choose to be down. I know the power of the mind.

On the following list are some, but not all, of the treatments and therapies that were part of Cheryl's regimen. Keep in mind that everyone with cancer, even the same kinds of cancer, needs to be evaluated personally and individually. The protocol for one type of cancer may not be beneficial for someone else with the identical type of cancer. The treatments and healing agents were administered at different times, in different doses, and for different reasons:

1. Acupuncture
2. Reiki
3. Prayer
4. Visualization
5. Recorded affirmations that put Cheryl to sleep peacefully every night.
6. Supplements to protect brain tissue, weaken the cancer, and enhance the immune system, approximately 30 per day.
7. Niacin
8. Germanium
9. Vitamin C
10. Vitamin E
11. Melatonin
12. St. John's wort
13. Soy genistein
14. Berberine
15. Glutathione
16. Quercetin
17. Alkylglycerois
18. Proanthocyanidins
19. Antioxidants
20. Omega-3 fatty acids
21. Siberian ginseng
22. Astragalus
23. Cat's claw
24. Mushroom extracts
25. Alca gliserols
26. 2Bromelain
27. A very healthy diet

For the first five years subsequent to my surgery, I did not have any sugar. Cutting out sugar in all forms is very important. Also: No white flour, no fried foods, no burgers, and virtually no red meat (maybe twice a year). Occasionally, I had organic turkey, wild salmon and tuna. I ate lots of fresh organic vegetables and greens, and allowed myself to have pizza once a month but only with fresh ingredients; not frozen, no pepperoni, no meat products on it, only vegetables. Just once a month.

In April of 2009, I found a lump on my right breast. Uggh, another shocker: Breast cancer. I decided to have a lumpectomy. Thank goodness there was no lymph node involvement, but I decided to engage in one round of chemo-therapy and some radiation. At this time, I became more rigorous with my nutritional regimen. After five years I had become less strict, but as a result of my newfound breast cancer, on top of my brain cancer, I cleaned up my diet even more.

I believe the different choices I made worked synergistically, to allow me to survive over 19 years now, and I have lived well. I do not believe the radiation alone would have allowed me to survive very long. After all, the doctors said the radiation was primarily palliative, not to mention the first doctor who said, "Get your affairs in order."

Today, I have an MRI once a year. I also take 25 supplements per day, plus melatonin before bedtime. Melatonin helps with chemo, radiation, and steroids. It combats inflammation and boosts the immune system. I also take IP6. This has been a prominent natural substance in my regimen to fight and keep cancer at bay. IP6 enhances cell-to-cell communication, induces cancer cell differentiation, enhances NK cell activity, and works well with chemotherapy.

Transformation and Pearls of Wisdom

I don't take the simple things in life for granted, anymore. I am grateful to stand, to walk, to take a shower, to be able to take a leisurely walk in my community and to enjoy the gorgeous views of the mountains by my house. I also love to go to the driving range. I love to ride my bike and throw my kayak into the back of my Subaru, which has over 200,000 miles on it, and go kayaking in the summer. I love to photograph nature. I am thankful to be here.

If I could tell anyone who was given a dire brain cancer diagnosis anything, I would say:

Don't give up hope. Don't let your doctor brainwash you into thinking you have no time left. You are not a statistic.

Also, if I could go back in time, one thing I would've changed was my eating habits. I would have eaten nutritional, beneficial food that helped every aspect of my health and avoided foods that are, ultimately, unhealthy for me, despite the fact that they tasted good. The lessons learned from the science of nutrition are tremendous.

Today, Cheryl is very active; she is not just a survivor. She enjoys a thriving life in Logan, Utah and continues to throw her kayak into the back of her Subaru, venture to regional waterways, and navigate her way down the beautiful rivers of Utah.

Cheryl has many, many miles to go, and treasures her time on earth every day.

SHARON

Sharon Dolan
Pancreatic Cancer
Diagnosed in 2009

"Just go home and live your life."
~Doctor's suggestion

Her Early Years Sharon and her two sisters grew up in Dunkirk, New York, close to Buffalo. Her father owned a collision shop and her mother was a stay-at-home mom. The early years were difficult with an upbringing that was dysfunctional due to her mom's drinking problems and the fact that her dad, who worked long hours, was often not at home.

Prior to high school graduation, Sharon and her sisters worked part time at their father's collision shop, sweeping the floors, helping sort paint cans and handling other tasks. Upon graduation in 1970, she worked at a sewing company known as M. Wile and Company for 20 years until the company closed.

Subsequently, Sharon attended nursing school where she became a licensed practical nurse, and later, a registered nurse, working over the years for a urologist, at a county home for the elderly, and caring for the disabled at a New York State disabled services organization.

Meet Sharon

The 1990s were very hard years. I was raising three children, and my mom and dad moved in with me in 1994. Mom had been suffering from Alzheimer's and died in 1995. Dad lived with me until 1999 when he passed away; he had lymph node cancer. I was also taking care of my aunt who lived nearby. She had a drinking problem and died of liver failure. Additionally, I was attending nursing school, gaining a lot of weight and got divorced in 1999. It was a very stressful time.

The early 2000s were not any easier. I remarried and now helped care for my mother-in-law. I always seemed to have lots of heartburn and consumed huge quantities of Tums. I continued to gain weight, but my doctor didn't say anything was seriously wrong, even when I had high blood pressure and got shingles. I dealt with a lot of stress in my job, and was always feeling very tired.

Toward the end of November 2008, my husband and I went on vacation to Key West, Florida. I had just completed my yearly physical with my primary doctor and received a clean bill of health. When I arrived in Florida I had a terrible itching sensation on the palms of my hands and the base of my feet. I had no appetite and couldn't eat. I felt full all the time and had lost 20 pounds within two weeks, even though I was not trying to lose weight! The itching became so severe I couldn't sleep; additionally, my hands and feet bled and developed scabs.

I returned to Buffalo on December 15th. I called my doctor from the Tampa airport and told him I was flying home and needed to see him as soon as possible. He told me to come in as soon as I arrived.

I stopped at my house to drop off my luggage and went straight to his office. He took one look at me and told me to turn around and pull my eyelids down as I looked in the mirror. To my surprise, my eyes looked like marbles and were yellow from jaundice. He then said there might be a cancer issue. He suspected a tumor on the head of my pancreas by the bile duct. He sent me to the hospital for an ultrasound.

My husband lost his first wife to lung cancer. She had died six months after diagnosis.

My husband fell apart, thinking I would die.

My doctor arranged for me to have an ERCP test (a diagnostic procedure that enables surgeons to examine pancreatic and bile ducts) on December 22nd. A scope was put down my throat into the first part of the small intestine to look at the biliary ducts. They found a tumor. He put a stent into the bile duct to open it, which caused my itching to become less severe. The bile had made me itch, terribly, as it was coming out through my skin.

You Have Pancreatic Cancer

I followed up on December 31st, 2008, with a surgeon who told me I had pancreatic cancer. It was adenocarcinoma of the head of the pancreas. He said I was very fortunate because I was a candidate for the Whipple procedure. He said I would die if I did not have the Whipple procedure and I might still die from the cancer, in the near future, even after having the procedure. He suggested that chemo might prolong my life.

At this time I was 56 years old and quickly determined there was no choice. I had the Whipple surgery on January 13th, 2009. It took six and a half hours. My doctor put two drains in. I remained in the hospital for 21 days and could not eat for 31 days after the surgery.

I was sent home and fed intravenously through a Peripherally Inserted Central Catheter (PICC line) line. My husband and I prepared the bag of nutrition each night with vitamins and insulin to run all night long. I had to wait for the drains to stop draining before I could eat any food. I constantly threw up green bile.

**I was getting very depressed about my ability to survive,
I did not think I would make it when I got home. I
felt this way for three weeks.**

I didn't think I would be able to walk or exercise again, but my husband got on my case and said, "You need to walk or you will be like this forever." He made me angry and I wanted to show him I could not do it.

Within two months after surgery I was walking two miles per day. When I could, I slowly began eating. I researched what I should eat and what I should avoid. I went on the Johns Hopkins online chat site, learned about and began taking Creon (an enzyme) to help me digest food. I also decided to eliminate sugar and milk from my diet.

In hindsight, from my early years until my cancer diagnosis, I had constantly consumed lots of sweets and Pepsi by the gallon. I had very poor eating habits.

Johns Hopkins Chat Room

Three months after surgery, I was talking to a woman online on the Johns Hopkins chat site. She strongly recommended I contact a woman who might help me, named Dr. Jeanne Wallace. Jeanne is the founder and director of Nutritional Solutions, which provides cutting-edge consultations with cancer patients, nationwide and internationally, about evidence-based dietary, nutritional and botanical support to complement conventional cancer care.

I called Jeanne's office and arranged for a one-hour phone consultation. Inclusive with the phone consultation, her firm put together a customized 125-page report, focused on me. The report had lots of specific nutritional information and included personalized recommendations of supplements to take each day, for my type of cancer. The report had rational explanations with supporting scientific studies, as to why each pill would be beneficial for my specific cancer issue.

Jeanne also recommended that I be tested for a variety of conditions, to take a closer look at my biochemistry because it would help her focus with relevant recommendations for me every three months. My cancer doctors refused to do these tests, but my primary doctor was very helpful and agreed to do so.

The tests Jeanne suggested included: C-reactive protein to detect internal inflammation; fasting blood glucose test to measure the amount of glucose, or sugar; fibrinogen to assess the viscosity of my blood; vitamin D test to measure the amount of vitamin D in my blood; copper test to monitor copper in my system that is believed to be the switch that turns on angiogenesis; TSH test which deals with thyroid as well as with some other cancer issues; iron-ferritin test which can be an indicator of certain cancer issues; and, a natural killer cell test which tests natural killer cell activity in my body.

Based upon the results of these tests, Jeanne tweaked my supplemental regimen with the goals of making my body inhospitable to cancer and doing everything I could to support my immune system. My doctors said I should not take any supplements or pills of any kind that they didn't prescribe, because they could work against the chemotherapy. However, Jeanne assured me, based upon her significant research, that her recommendations would not work against the chemo. I chose to follow Jeanne's recommendations and did not tell my conventional doctors about her supplementation regimen.

I had four weeks of chemotherapy, followed by 31 radiation treatments, then three more months of chemo. The chemotherapy was gemcitabine and Xeloda. I diligently followed Jeanne's nutritional and supplementation recommendations taking 62 pills per day, throughout my chemo and radiation treatments. I had very few side effects, unlike many others who suffer terrible side effects. My radiologist stated he wished all his patients were able to handle the radiation as well as me.

In January of 2010, I was down to 116 pounds and I was not trying to lose weight. Despite the weight loss, I was actually feeling pretty good.

Then, two years after the Whipple procedure I noticed a lump in my groin. I had hernia surgery and, then again, lost eight more pounds during the next three months. By June of 2011, I lost another eight pounds and was now down to 100 pounds. I noticed a lot of greasy stool, bloating and gas. At this point, I had another serious scare.

Spots on Lungs and Liver, and Precipitous Weight Loss
In June of 2011, my doctor found two spots on my lungs from contrast CT scans. My doctors and I assumed the cancer had recurred and metastasized.

We repeated the scans a month later and they had disappeared, but now the doctors found two spots on my liver. My husband and I moved to Florida at this time, because I wanted to be closer to my daughter and granddaughter. Within two weeks after arriving in Florida I had an ultrasound (in September, 2011) and a CT scan with contrast. To my doctor's surprise, the spots on the liver had also disappeared.

I should mention, that before my Whipple surgery, and after the second surgery, I asked my doctors several times, "How long do I have to live?"

They never gave me an exact time frame, but continually said, "Just go home and live your life." I know they felt my situation was quite grave and did not believe I would be alive much longer.

In March of 2012, I was down to 90 pounds. My doctors did not know why. They did an endoscopy and found a large ulcer. Normally, these ulcers are treated with medicine, but it was too big to be treated effectively with medication. Therefore, surgery became an option. One of my doctors said, "No, don't do surgery. Take drugs." He repeated the endoscopy procedure a month later, and after this second procedure, his nurse practitioner said, "You probably won't be able to have surgery, because you're too weak." I was now down to 85 pounds and I was very weak. With my precipitous and continuing weight loss, I did not think I would live much longer, but I had to do something.

Understanding the risks, as a nurse, I talked my surgical doctor into doing the surgery, fully knowledgeable that it was questionable if I would even make it through surgery. The surgery I had was called the Roux-en-Y. It lasted six hours. I had a continuing fever and was in the ICU and hospital, for eight days. When I went home I was fed through a feeding tube for five weeks. It took a full year to gain any measurable weight.

Transformation and Pearls of Wisdom

Despite my serious bout with pancreatic cancer, my large ulcer and my extreme weight loss, I was able to regain my health. Five things were critical in my quest to get better: First, my faith in God; second, researching and getting educated about all the different science based options that might help, conventional and alternative; third, asking lots of questions of my doctors; fourth, keeping track of every laboratory and medical test I had; and fifth, learning why my doctors recommended these tests. I became diligent about doing these things.

> **You must have hope. I told two close friends, both in their 50s, about Jeanne Wallace, but they refused to call her. They died. It is a lot of work, changing your lifestyle, taking the supplements, and it is not easy, but it is absolutely worth it to live.**

You need to take care of yourself. Listen to your body, pay attention to changes and document those changes carefully so you can provide information to your doctor. Every day is a gift, especially when I get to see my grandchildren. I quilt; I look at beautiful things in life—sunrises, sunsets and flowers. Family is important— you are not here forever, so enjoy life, be happy. Make memories for them.

> **My surgeon said I had a very strong will to live. He and my other doctors said, "People with pancreatic cancer usually die within three years." He also said, "I don't have anyone living this long with this disease."**

People looked at me with fear when I was down to 85 pounds. I overheard them say, "She won't live." My surgeon cannot explain how I am alive. He said, "It is a God thing."

Everyone who has cancer needs someone like Jeanne Wallace to do the serious research, to find additional complementary medical options that are right, specifically, for you. Today, I still work with Jeanne Wallace and follow most of her recommendations regarding nutrition and supplementation.

Exercise, positive attitude, prayer, nutritional food, science-based supplements, an accumulation of a variety of things saved my life.

I also attend a cancer support group and according to my research, this type of support can extend a patient's life. There is a doctor at each group meeting, every week, to answer patient questions.

I would not be here without Jeanne Wallace's science-based guidance and support; I would not be here if it was not for my doctors, and I would not be here if was not for God.

Sharon ended the interview by saying: "Never give up until your last breath."

JOHN

John S. Strauss
Melanoma
Diagnosed in 1991

"There are not any successful treatments here.
You may want to consider participating in a study."
~Two oncologists at a major cancer center

His Early Years John grew up on a dairy farm in Wisconsin, in a mostly Roman Catholic town, with six siblings: four brothers and two sisters. His upbringing was comprised predominantly of "milking a lot of cows," working hard on the farm and going to church. In high school he spent a couple of years in seminary, graduating in 1962.

John left the farm behind and attended the University of Wisconsin as an electrical engineering major. During his junior year he was a foreign exchange student in Monterrey, Mexico, at an institution generally known as "the MIT of Mexico."

After college graduation, he married in 1968 and found a job with Honeywell in the Twin Cities. After a couple of years John's career took him to Motorola in Schaumberg, Illinois, where he worked for 13 years.

Diagnosis In October of 1991, John was 47 years old. He went to his doctor for his annual physical and asked him to take a look at something on his right side, above the waist, towards his back. John described it as, "something the size of an eraser, but not that high off the skin, perhaps elevated one-eighth of an inch."

Meet John

My doctor said, "We need to have this checked out." He arranged a meeting with another doctor who excised the skin abnormality and then had it biopsied. He had removed the tumor and some surrounding flesh. The results came back on October 23rd, and my doctor said, "We need to do more."

A year earlier, the doctor took a look at this same area and said the skin abnormality was "no big deal," so I just assumed at that time, it was nothing to be concerned about. He was so wrong.

Surgery and Diagnosis

On November 10th, 1991, I had surgery that entailed a large incision around that area to remove any suspicious cancerous cells. The doctor also looked under my arm, on the same side, and took out approximately 12 lymph nodes. The doctors were concerned that the cancer might have traveled.

Lo and behold, approximately half of the 12 lymph nodes were malignant. This was not good, especially since the cancer had traveled much farther from its original site.

I was in the hospital for a couple of days after surgery. I had expressed my anger at my doctor the day before I was dismissed from the hospital. This was the doctor who said, a year before, that it was "no big deal." As a result, he decided to get me a different doctor to follow up and treat me.

Dire Prognosis

My new doctor arranged for me to meet an oncologist. This doctor had nothing promising to tell me. He said, "There are not any successful treatments for your type of cancer." He then proceeded to send me to two young oncologists at a major medical center. They essentially told me the same thing: "You might want to consider participating in a study for your cancer." I would be thrown into a lottery. I would either be given a placebo or placed in another group to get one type of injection of drugs, or in yet another group to get two injections.

They had nothing to offer except this study. I asked them about statistics. I wanted to know what my chances were. As an engineer, I wanted to see numbers. They showed me stats that demonstrated that most people are dead inside of two years, approximately 80 percent.

I thought I would not make it to 50 years of age.

I had been attending an Executive MBA Program at Northwestern University paid for by my employer. Although I had now completed half of the course work, my doctors discouraged me from continuing the program. They felt, due to my prognosis and condition, that it would be too difficult to continue.

Hope from Keith Block, M.D.

I was not ready to give up. The day after I was dismissed from the major medical center, a friend of mine who knew of my situation said, "John, go see Dr. Block. Tell him you know me and get an appointment."

> John was not ready to go home and wait for his cancer to progressively destroy his health, despite the fact his doctors impliedly offered no hope, since they did not prescribe any medicine or craft any type of protocol.

My friend informed me that Dr. Block's treatments were a bit "out of the box," but I should not hesitate and I should call him right away.

When you are desperate, you become open to anything, especially when your doctors are implying that you won't be here much longer.

I will never forget my meeting with Dr. Block. I went in with no hope, whatsoever; no one had any good suggestions at all. He talked to me for 45 minutes, one-on-one. He really cared, even though he had just met me. He had a program that offered hope that might benefit me. For the most part, his message was, "We will get your body healthy and strong, and your body will solve your health problems."

Dr. Block and his team put together a specific nutritional diet for me. I discussed the cancer-fighting diet with his dietician for quite a while. This program was specific regarding breakfast, lunch and dinner, as well as what I should eat and avoid eating.

The transition was easy for me, because I felt this regimen could help me beat my cancer. My level of determination and motivation was very high. I followed directions very carefully. Mostly plant-based foods made up the diet, including all kinds of berries. Meat of any kind was discouraged, but ocean fish was acceptable. I was strongly discouraged from drinking any alcohol or coffee. I was also encouraged to eat organic food as much as possible. Today, I am 99 percent vegan.

I needed to lose weight. I lost 42 pounds in six months through aerobic exercise and jogging. I also took approximately 20 supplements per day including various vitamins and herbs. I embraced Dr. Block's protocol for approximately five years. I did not have any radiation or chemotherapy. I continue to stay committed to most of the program, but have weaned off some of the supplements. I live in the moment.

During the early part of my protocol I attended a cancer support group, 12 meetings in all. I found the group to be a good experience, but 12 meetings were enough. You hear too many horror stories in these groups.

On the religious or spiritual front, I have not been a practicing Catholic for a long time. I am a Buddhist. I meditate daily. I have done a lot of reading about Buddhism.

I knew a lot of people who had metastatic melanoma like myself. All of them are dead.

They did not know Dr. Block or they refused to see him, despite my strong encouragement for them to do so. It has been over 25 years since the doctors said, "There are no successful treatments for your type of cancer." I am here because of Dr. Block, absolutely, one hundred percent.

Transformation and Pearls of Wisdom

I have been through a lot of emotional, scary times since my diagnosis. Cancer puts everything in perspective about what is important in life.

> **Before diagnosis, compared to after diagnosis, my atti-tude changed about material things. In my former life, I was a corporate star, a hotshot executive. That is not important anymore.**

I now see my kids and grandkids. I now have more time to meditate, read and study all kinds of things about the world. I recommend meditation to everyone. I believe it is very helpful. People should not be afraid of their minds.

People eat too much food. They throw poison in their bodies. There is a lot of poison in grocery stores. Stay away from it.

Statistics don't tell you anything about what will happen to you. They work for groups, not individuals. They can't tell you about any particular person or a specific issue.

> **When I walk around Chicago and see people on the street I ask myself, "Why aren't they taking care of themselves?" Surround yourself with people who want to be healthy.**

In our culture, we wait until there is a crisis before we act. If I had been part of a health program like Dr. Block's before 1991, maybe things would have been different.

DIANE

Diane Klenke
Pancreatic Cancer
Diagnosed in 2004

"I would give you, maybe tops, three months to live.
We can arrange for hospice care, if you like."
~Doctor's prognosis at a major Midwest cancer center

Her Early Years Stress was like a constant companion for Diane from a very early age. It permeated most aspects of her youth and affected the entire family. Growing up in the Midwest under the Christian guidance of her caring mother, Diane's discovery of a malignancy in her body happened in her adult years, thanks to another illness that was unrelated to cancer.

Meet Diane

I grew up in a crazy world. My mom was supportive, but came from a poor background. My dad was an abusive alcoholic. My brother was 2½ when my parents adopted him, and I was 7. We were raised Christian by my mom and are very close to God and Jesus Christ. Our reliance in our relationship with God helped us get through the stupid things we endured with my dad. He would sit with guns in the living room and point them at us and say, "One of these days everyone is going to die around here." I think that is where I began to develop inner strength. I would stand up to him throughout my childhood to protect my mom and brother, and made him leave the house when he tried to kill my brother.

I began working at an early age to help with the finances, food and things we needed for school. My brother, mom and I loved the outdoors, wild-life and nature. We spent lots of time together fishing, gardening, chasing butterflies and healing small, injured animals. I have always been very active; running, walking the dog, gardening, doing lawn work, playing volleyball and enjoying cross-country skiing. I would much rather work hard outside than do vacuuming.

Dad smoked cigars and chewed them, but he was not allowed to do it in the house. He really wasn't home very much. He was out drinking, chasing other women, and spending a lot of time in bars.

I was a straight-A student and was hoping to attend medical school, but there was no money to do so. My brother joined the Marine Corps after graduation, and he continued to send mom money after I was married.

To put it mildly, we had a very stressful life, but I wasn't going to let it defeat me. My dad's parents were divorced early in life. Grandma and Grandpa were drunks too. My grandpa died of pancreatic cancer when I was about 17.

Thank Goodness for Gas

Diane did not have any specific signs of cancer while growing up. One Friday in February of 2004, while working at an insurance office in Green Bay, Wisconsin, the entire office staff came down with a nasty virus. Everyone was so sick they went to the local emergency room. Diane said she had bloating symptoms and "horrible gas pains, which were not passing." She had known of someone who had died of a stomach aneurism and said, "I was scared and went to the ER. I was doubled over in pain."

She had blood work and was given a shot. The bloating was relieved and Diane was sent home. She was told it was a virus. When her blood work came back from the lab, she was told she had high liver enzymes. Her family had a history of gall bladder problems, so it was suggested that she follow up with her family doctor and have an ultrasound to check for gallstones.

The following Thursday, while undergoing the ultrasound at the local hospital, Diane noticed the tech had a perplexed look on his face, but he didn't disclose his suspicions to her. The hospital called her doctor who then suggested that she "spend the night for more tests," but he didn't tell her about possible concerns.

After undergoing more tests, Diane visited with her doctor the next day. He said, "You have a very large tumor in your pancreas, three tumors in your liver and tumors around your portal vein." These results were evident from the various tests and the CT scan. The doctor did not know, definitively, if they were malignant, but they were very suspicious and troubling.

Get Your Affairs in Order

A few days later, Diane had an appointment with a surgeon in Green Bay. She recalled the doctor's exact words: "This appears to be a widespread cancer. You might as well go home and get your affairs in order. You are inoperable and don't have long for this world."

This pronouncement was less than two weeks after her visit to the emergency room. Diane's husband cried for days.

As a result of her troubled upbringing, Diane had learned to become a fighter. She was determined and would not go down without doing everything in her power to beat the cancer. There was no time to waste.

Medical records were immediately sent to a well-known hospital in Minnesota. Within a week she traveled to the hospital for a meeting with an oncologist and surgeon. Her liver and pancreas were biopsied. The dire diagnosis of the Green Bay doctor was confirmed: Malignant cancer.

The oncologist and surgical oncologist said: "Your chances of survival are maybe one percent. I would give you maybe, tops, three months to live. We can arrange for hospice care, if you like." Diane was astounded. She said, "No, I feel fine." She then decided to seek further advice from a different healthcare institution dedicated to fighting cancer. She sent them her medical records.

They could only offer a clinical trial and it might be a blind trial, and I said no. A blind trial only offers half of the participants the actual experimental drug; the other half receive a placebo. Both sides are "blind" as to who is treated with the real drug, so there is serious risk in "blind studies," whether or not a patient is getting a potentially beneficial treatment.

A Green Bay oncology group was willing to treat Diane with chemotherapy, despite the fact their prognosis was quite grave, at best. They said, "Eat anything you want, you need calories. Ice cream; whatever you want."

I responded, "I have cut out sugar and dairy. I am now taking vitamin C supplements." The Green Bay doctors said, "We will not treat you if you take vitamins. It will interfere with the chemo."

The doctors did not appreciate Diane's feisty attitude, her questions, her desire to find other options and her refusal to accept her so-called fate. Pompously, according to Diane, the Green Bay doctor said, "Lady, you are terminal." Diane indicated strongly that this "omniscient attitude" prevailed at the other cancer centers as well.

My chemo treatment was set for Monday.

New Hope

Prior to starting chemo treatments with the Green Bay doctors, Diane's daughter's father-in-law told her that he knew of a patient who experienced great success with the Block Center for Integrative Cancer Treatment. On the Internet, Diane looked up Dr. Keith Block, the founder and owner of the Center, and liked what she saw. She called Dr. Block's clinic and immediately made an appointment. In the meantime, she postponed her chemo treatments.

Diane was feeling a new sense of optimism after her visit with Dr. Block. He said, "I think we can alter this cancer." No promises of a cure or long-term remission, but at least some hope that was offered versus the no-hope prospects echoed by the other doctors.

He said, "We can start chemo if you pass a MUGA test." This test examines the heart for pre-existing conditions, prior to chemo and/ or the impact of chemo.

Dr. Block told me:

"The immune system is like an army. We need to strengthen the army to stop the progression of cancer. At the same time, we need to strengthen the body."

Dr. Block continued, "Nutrition and the appropriate supplements will help strengthen and protect the body from the toxic effects of chemotherapy. We need to starve the tumors as well. You need to cut out sugar, red meat, dairy, and many other foods."

Chronomodulated Chemotherapy The chemo treatments given to Diane were chronomodulated. These treatments are given at specific times of the day (thus the word "chrono" as in chronology), when cancer cells are most vulnerable. To my knowledge, the Block Center for Integrative Cancer Treatment is the only cancer center or clinic in the U.S. that uses a chronomodulated technique. However, according to Dr. Block, this technique is used in over 40 cancer centers throughout Europe.

Diane was subjected to various tests to determine the optimum time when she should be given her treatments. Contrary to many conventional doctors, but in accordance with many integrative doctors, Dr. Block believes that certain vitamins and/or supplements can mitigate the toxicity of chemotherapy.

Immediately prior to being treated with chemotherapy, Dr. Block gave me a significant infusion of vitamins and specific supplements to help the healthy cells survive the harsh impact of the chemo, and to maximize the potency of the chemo, without subjecting me to potentially harsh side effects.

At the start, Diane was given one particular chemotherapy drug for six months. Diagnostic tests indicated the tumor in the pancreas stopped growing, but it did not shrink. There was even better news regarding the tumors in her liver: by the third month, the cancer in her liver was shrinking. After six months, the tumors in her liver had virtually disappeared!

During the first six months, Diane was given her chemo at certain times of day, primarily early morning, with a portable pump. During months six through 12, she had a fanny pack style pump that sent a combination of two chemotherapy drugs into her body at specific times of the day. She also had a double port located just above her heart on the left side of her chest. Even while receiving chemo from the fanny pack, she was also given certain vitamins and supplements just prior to receiving her chemo.

Every day, Diane ingested between 50 to 80 pills—specific vitamins and supplements—tailored for her condition, prescribed by Dr. Block. After 20 months, Diane stopped the chronomodulated chemotherapy treatments. However, she did not stop taking multiple supplements, nor did she stop engaging in her newfound nutritional lifestyle. After 20 months, she continued to have regular check-ups and scans to ascertain whether the cancer had come back.

I never missed work while going through my chemo treatments.

Additionally, I stuck to my diet and took all of my supplements.

**I had a great motivation to live, and I never really
feared death. You want to live? Just do it!**

I am a toughie. I ignored the doctors who said I would die. I just needed the right path. I prayed that God would lead me to the right people, to lead me through this journey.

Dr. Block told me a few years ago, "I saw a determination in you and a willingness to follow the program. I thought you would be here at least five years after the diagnosis." Today, there is only dead tissue, residual necrosis in the pancreas.

Mind-Body Visualization Penny Block, Ph.D., is the co-founder and executive director of the Block Cancer Center. She also has an expertise in behavioral medicine and psychosocial oncology. She was very helpful to Diane regarding psychological issues.

Additionally, a visualization expert at the Center told Diane, "I want you to visualize, numerous times per day, and definitely before bed, that the tumor is shrinking. I want you to visualize that a Pac-Man is eating the tumor, or visualize that the tumor is shrinking. Do this 30 times per day."

Current Diet Diane has not deviated from her strict cancer-fighting diet ever since she began working with the Block Cancer Center.

I eat lots of vegetables, fruits, whole grains, beans, nuts, lots of spinach and avocado, and I drink almond milk and green tea. I also eat fish about three times per week, and ground turkey once per week. I do not eat anything with sugar. Red meat, fried foods, and dairy are dirty words to me. I do not eat anything with white flour.

Transformation and Pearls of Wisdom

I asked Diane, "What would you tell someone with a dire prognosis?"

Don't believe it; fight. Ask questions about treatments, lots of questions. Why are you doing this test, why this treatment, how will it affect me?

I also asked, "How does someone find a doctor like Dr. Keith Block?"

Most people don't want to upset the family. They just go with the local doctor and do whatever they say. Families ask, "If doctors say, 'It is over,' why waste money?" I was lucky to find Dr. Block, but you need to do research. Something all cancer patients need to do is get many copies of their records, regarding everything. You need to move quickly; you must communicate with doctors and be proactive.

The Green Bay oncology group became curious, in hindsight, about my treatment. Now, they are shocked that I am still alive. They have become more open-minded and send their tough cases to Dr. Block.

You must make your body inhospitable to cancer. Diet, supplements, chemotherapy; the way Dr. Block does it. Exercise and prayer are also big reasons why I am here today.

Dr. Block told me:

> **"Don't ever consider yourself cured of cancer; you must stay with the program. You may always have cancer cells that could cause problems again, even if you are 10 years down the road. You must change your life."**

In an Interview with CNN, Diane Klenke spoke with Dr. Sanjay Gupta and Dr. Keith Block. Following is the transcript, verbatim, of that interview which aired on CNN on June 24th, 2006 (including grammatical errors):

GUPTA: Two years ago, the peaceful life Diane Klenke was accustomed to, began to slowly fall apart. It started with mild discomfort in her abdomen then...

DIANE KLENKE, CANCER PATIENT: I was doubled over in pain. I was just miserable.

GUPTA: She was rushed to the hospital. And hours later, doctors were still pouring over her case.

KLENKE: But I said tell me what's going on. Well, we see something we want to check out further.

GUPTA: The news was grim. Diane's pancreas and liver had been hijacked by cancer. One tumor was the size of a grapefruit. Doctors told Klenke that not even chemotherapy could help her. She had mere months to live. You're thinking at that time was what? I mean, were you thinking OK, you know, maybe it is time to get my affairs in order.

KLENKE: I wasn't willing to give up yet. I thought I've got too much to live for. I've got—my daughter was pregnant. And I had another daughter just engaged. And I thought I want to be here.

GUPTA: With few options left, Klenke tried something called chronotherapy.

DR. KEITH BLOCK, BLOCK CENTER FOR INTEGRATIVE CANCER TREATMENT: Chronotherapy is all about timing. Nine genes are the molecular timekeeper for our entire physiology. Just like flowers open up, you know, when it's light out in the morning and close up at night, we have entire physiological rhythms that are being adjusted through the day and night and through the seasons.

GUPTA: With chronotherapy, patients are quizzed about their habits, sleep patterns, diet, exercise—all things that impact the body's internal clock. Chemo drugs are pumped in on a precise timetable based on that information, synchronized to the body's internal rhythms. So instead of a daily dose at say 10:00 a.m. every day, Diane received chemotherapy while she slept, when her healthy cells were dormant and her cancer cells were active.

BLOCK: We can actually time drugs so that they'll diminish a lot of the side effects. And at the same time, it can also boost the effectiveness of the therapies.

GUPTA: Timing is not just for treating cancer. It can also be used to help diagnose heart disease and stroke. Using our internal clocks as a guide, we know now that stress hormones soar in the morning, as does blood pressure in the afternoon. Those fluctuations may explain why heart attacks are so common in the morning and strokes during midday. Chronotherapy helps when doctors can time blood pressure readings so they're measured throughout the day, instead of just once. Using internal cues, we may one day predict stroke.

EARL BAKKEN, NORTH HAWAII COMMUNITY HOSPITAL: So when they have a normal blood pressure, when they go in to have it examined in the morning, but may have—be hypertensive in the afternoon but never get measured in the afternoon.

GUPTA: Chronotherapy is used in a handful of medical facilities. It is now used to treat depression, sleep disorders and asthma. It seems simple. We're not talking about changing the world here. We're not talking about new therapies. We're not talking about billions of dollars of drug research. We're talking about using a clock. Why isn't everyone doing this?

BLOCK: It's not convenient for the doctor to work around the patient's schedule. They really have to change their entire medical center to work around the patient's schedule instead of working really around the medical center's schedule.

GUPTA: Timing caused Diane's grapefruit size tumor to shrink to the size of a kidney bean. And...

KLENKE: They looked at my liver and said, "Hey, the liver tumors are gone."

GUPTA: A lot of people say that's all quackery. You know what....

KLENKE: Oh, absolutely not. Absolutely not.

GUPTA: You're living proof that it isn't?

KLENKE: I'm living proof that it isn't.

GUPTA: For now, Klenke is relishing her new lease on life and being around for her family. Dr. Sanjay Gupta, CNN, reporting.

JULIA

Julia Chiappetta
Breast Cancer
Diagnosed in 2000

"If you go with a natural protocol, you will die."
~Doctor's opinion

Her Early Years Julia grew up in an idyllic setting. She attended a highly respected school system in Greenwich, Connecticut, played the cello, the guitar, and was very involved in sports.

She was surrounded by a big, loving Italian family that came together frequently at family gatherings. Her grandparents from the "old country," grew vegetables in their backyard.

At college, Julia was bored and wanted to get on with her life. She left college and found a position with American Express where she hit the fast track, sometimes working 80 hours per week.

At American Express, Julia discovered that she had unique social and organizational skills. After gaining valuable experience, she decided to leave American Express to start her own firm, where she specialized in organizing events and parties for high-end clientele. She was living the fast life, with designer clothes and first-class hotels. Organizing elite, glamorous events, she traveled the globe as a highly paid meeting planner. She worked and played hard on stressful trips abroad, "giving her all" to satisfy her high-end clientele. Health was secondary; clients and "the high life" came first. Julia was burning the candle at both ends.

Meet Julia

I was working six days per week. When I had the time, I was involved in extreme athletic training. I was always on the run, literally running six miles per day. I was becoming fatigued more quickly than usual. Fatigue was my symptom. I rationalized that since I was working 80-hour weeks, traveling the globe, that anyone would be tired. However, looking back I believe my fatigue was not just a symptom, but also a contributor to my breast cancer.

Discovering the Lump

In December of 1999, I had a physical exam with my doctor. I was always good about getting my annual mammogram and physical. Nothing showed up. In early 2000, I made several trips to Europe. I became more fatigued. Then, one Sunday evening in early March, while doing my monthly self-examination, I felt a minor lump on the outer edge of my breast. It was different, like nothing I had ever felt before. I was a bit panicked, so I met with my gynecologist the very next day, and had a new mammogram.

After receiving the results, the doctor said, "No problem; there is nothing wrong. Come back in six months." I said, "No, something is wrong here." My doctor sat me down and again said, "It is no big deal." I wanted a biopsy and after continued contentious discussion, she reluctantly agreed to do a biopsy the next day. The doctor and her staff made me feel like I didn't know what I was talking about. They made me feel like I was a "bothersome, pain-in-the-neck patient."

The Doctor's Sobering Diagnosis and Prognosis

The very next day, my doctor said, "I want to apologize to you. I just learned a lesson: I need to listen to my patients much more closely. They know better than I about what is going on in their bodies." Then she said, "You have an aggressive breast cancer. We need to do something about this right now." I had an infiltrating ductal carcinoma, Stage 2. My doctor said, "You need a mastectomy, preferably a double mastectomy, then radiation and probably chemotherapy, followed by Tamoxifen."

This was the most terrifying, shocking thing I'd ever heard. My first thought was, "I am going to die." I knew I did not want to do chemo, I had five friends who had died from chemo treatment; slow, painful deaths, not from the cancer, but from the treatment.

My feeling was, and is, that we are so antiquated in this country. All we do is cut (surgery), burn (radiation) and poison (chemotherapy).

I told my doctor, "I am just going to go with a natural protocol." She responded, "If you go with a natural protocol, you will die."

Call to Action

I had a friend, a scientist, who said he wanted to help me find the best treatments or therapies to help me beat this cancer. Inspired by my research, with my friend's help, I threw out everything with chemicals in my house. I cleaned the closets and shelves of anything I felt might be toxic. I threw out everything that contained hormones, antibiotics and toxins like lead, parabens, and sulfates that may have contributed to my cancer. I tossed out all of my food, my makeup, shampoos and my microwave oven. I converted to a raw, organic vegan diet. I got rid of my beloved bread, cheese, pasta and chicken. I also added specific nutrients and supplements, including juicing three times per day with vegetables and greens, including wheat grass to detox my body of the build-up of junk over time. I began to use only organic products with natural ingredients. I read everything I could get my hands on regarding natural treatments and therapies.

Also, my prayer life is very important to me; I leaned on this component for inner support and comfort. Within two weeks, I felt much better and stronger.

I felt this would not be a death sentence. My inner confidence with this path gave me the courage to stand up to the doctors, even though I was crying frequently.

They were unsupportive. Their words resonated inside me: "You are wrong. It is not going to work. You are going to die." Many of my friends, clients and colleagues said, "Are you crazy?" Regardless, I really was at peace with my decision.

Second Opinion

Still, I needed help. I started to look for second opinions. Everyone has an opinion, and most people believe their opinion is best. I needed to speak to people who were supportive and knowledgeable.

I heard about a cancer institution known as MD Anderson, probably the largest and most well known institution of its kind in the U.S. I flew to Houston, Texas to meet with two doctors there.

They were very thorough. They carefully read my file, learned about every aspect of my history and worked with me, collaboratively, to implement a plan to deal with my cancer. Still I had to deal with the recommendations of my doctor in Connecticut who recommended a mastectomy or double mastectomy. The doctors at MD Anderson recommended a lumpectomy. I had the surgery in May 2000. My margins were clean.

I was continually eating healthy raw foods, specific supplements, and wheatgrass—and implementing other natural treatments. My tumor markers were now, subsequent to surgery, in the normal range. I attribute this to my healthy lifestyle changes.

Contrary to popular opinion, 15 percent of the patients just do the natural protocol at MD Anderson. I was a very engaged advocate for myself; I took care of myself. Although MD Anderson recommended radiation and Tamoxifen post surgery, I decided not to go down that path. I felt surgery was enough. My blood work looked great after a few months.

Making Changes

You must leave behind the negative people who could drag you down. I left behind my 80-hour workweek and my six-figure income. The protocol must be about serious changes. Most people do chemo and radiation and go back to the same stressful lives and poor habits—and have recurrences or worse.

**You must be steadfast in staying with
a strict, healthy program.**

Other well-known cancer institutions would not be supportive of my decision. I was happy MD Anderson worked with me and my unconventional, natural approach. During the first two years after my first visit to MD Anderson I returned every four months for scans and a complete checkup. Since then, I have returned every six months for blood work, ultrasounds, and to check my tumor markers.

I also see Dr. George Wong in New York City. George is a Chinese medicine expert and I take his herbs every day. Additionally, I take 30 different other herbs and botanicals per day.

Bigger Changes

I was now done with my flurry of activity, with the initial treatments. I decided to move to Florida. I needed a change from the daily life, the rat race of the New York metropolitan area. I took a consulting job in Fort Lauderdale, now making one-third of what I was making in New York, but I was near the ocean, more relaxed and loving it. I needed a different approach to life; it is hard to make big changes like this, but it was great. In Connecticut I existed to pay my significant bills, to support my lifestyle. My life was not about the things that are important. We need to bring joy into our lives, every day.

**The career became the all-important thing in my life. I
needed to change everything in my life, and I did.**

Today, I am very focused about what I put into my body, at every meal. I take supplements that bring real health value. My environment is clean and I shop for local organic produce. My diet is virtually the same as 16 years ago, after I was diagnosed.

Honestly, approximately once per month I may deviate a bit and eat something I shouldn't. I am not perfect, but I am reminded of this as my body does not feel great afterwards. I fast occasionally, and just drink alkaline water with lemons or sometimes just carrots and beet juice. I detox quarterly. Once per year I do colonics.

Transformation and Pearls of Wisdom

Julia radically transformed herself in so many ways. She became more emotionally grounded and at peace with herself; she changed her perspective about what was important in life. Julia became a very strong advocate, every day, for her health.

This experience made me realize that I lost sight of who Julia was. I started feeling pressure in high school. Before that, I loved nature, to write, to play in the garden, to play the cello. As time goes on you feel the pressures of being successful, of making money, and you measure yourself by financial success and status. I had to purge myself of all the junk I accumulated over the years. A layer of healing took place when I went through this process. This has, in a way, been a gift to me. I was too absorbed with my world.

There is no going back to the old Julia. I was not truly happy inside with the person I had become. When you are faced with a diagnosis of cancer, the designer clothes don't matter, the fancy parties don't matter anymore. You must release all the junk from your life.

Don't be afraid. Don't allow doctors or the establishment to pressure you. You need to have a higher power, whether it is meditation, God or whatever. This is not a death sentence. It is a lifelong commitment to staying well.

I don't consider myself a survivor. I am healed, I believe my body is strong and I don't believe I will get sick again. I don't like the word remission, but I must take care of myself every day to consciously keep my body strong and make it feel good.

I work part-time now and earn much less than what I used to earn. But I have never felt more free. I have learned to live with so much less. Having a big house and a closet full of beautiful shoes and clothes means nothing when your doctor says the word "cancer."

Cancer did not kill me. It woke me up to who I really am and empowered me to make my own choices. Was it a gift? Yes, it helped me find the real me.

NICHOLAS

Nicholas Steiner, M.D.
Melanoma
Diagnosed in 1964

"You should do chemo directly into your spinal fluid;
it might get you two to three more months."
~Doctor in New York City

His Early Years Nicholas Steiner was born in Germany. He immigrated
to the United States when he was three months old. He graduated
from New Lincoln School in New York City and subsequently graduated from Yale University with a liberal arts degree, then attended
and graduated from the medical school at Wayne State University.

As a boy, Nicholas lived close to the beaches on the South Shore
of Long Island, New York, and by his own admission, spent much
too much time at the beach, unprotected, exposed to the sun.

Meet Nicholas

In 1964, I was 29 years old and midway through the first year of my medical
residence at Roosevelt Hospital in New York City. Late one afternoon while
searching some films in the x-ray department, Bertha the technician stood next
to me and said, "Watcha got there, Doc, a beauty mark?"

Dr. Steiner assumed the two or three millimeter-sized dark brown
spot had probably always been there. He thought it was no big deal.

A few days later I was about to examine an elderly patient who raised one hand as if to swat me and said, "Hold still, Doc, you've got a fly on your neck!" That did it. The next day I paged Dr. Llowyd Ballantyne, one of Roosevelt's plastic surgeons and asked whether he might be able to excise a little skin growth that had come to my attention. He did, and it took only a couple of minutes to remove it.

Melanoma: "Why me?"

One week later, my beeper went off. It was Dr. Ballantyne. He said, "It turns out to have been a melanoma, but fortunately I think we got all of it." I felt like I had just been clobbered with a sledgehammer. Melanoma? I was 29 years old. Why me?

Dr. Ballantyne said we could be very aggressive and, "Go for a bilateral radical neck dissection and a sternal-splitting, bilateral mediastinal cleanout, but it is probably not appropriate or even necessary. You're almost certainly cured."

In 1968, Dr. Steiner entered private practice specializing in internal medicine with a cardio sub-specialty. His practice grew; life was good. In 1970, however, he had another melanoma removed from his arm. He thought it was nothing to worry about, just another minor procedure.

Time flew. It was 1980 and Dr. Steiner had been enjoying a comfortable life. Happily married, he was living in the affluent suburbs with two wonderful children.

Melanoma Recurrence

One night, while I was brushing my teeth, my wife spotted something unusual behind my right knee. I ignored it, assuming it was nothing. I noticed it again three weeks later, and at her urging I had it looked at and biopsied. This time it was a more sinister and deeper melanoma. The following week, I was admitted to Roosevelt Hospital for a wide excision and skin graft, taken from elsewhere on my leg. I chose to think that once again, the lesion's removal would result in a cure.

As it turned out, others in my life were deeply worried and not without reason. I was in denial.

Metastasis One day, during the spring of 1983, Dr. Steiner visited Dr. Albert Attia, his internist, for a routine checkup. He had been feeling well since the removal of his nodular melanoma, three years before.

Part way through my doctor's usual careful physical exam, his fingers lingered in my right groin area. Then came the thunderbolt, "Nick, were you aware of having a couple of lymph nodes here? They're small, but definitely enlarged and quite firm." In an instant my own fingers confirmed the findings, and I knew.

Christ! No doubt about it. I knew I had metastatic cancer.

I now needed to take serious action. Shortly thereafter, I had surgery at Memorial Sloan Kettering, a radical lymph node dissection of the groin.

A few months after my dissection of the groin, I had two additional recurrences in the lymph nodes of the groin, each necessitating a brief hospitalization and surgery. With each recurrence the hope of a prolonged remission grew fainter.

In September of 1984, I sold my practice, which was becoming quite stressful, especially with my health concerns. Almost immediately after selling my practice, I was readmitted to Memorial for abdominal surgery. A lymph node in my pelvis had shown up on a routine CT scan and was excised by Dr. Brennan.

In February of 1985, I attended a medical conference in Sugarbush, Vermont. I brought the family, and we enjoyed a fun vacation combining it with the medical meetings I attended. Within one hour of returning to New York, I leaned up against the kitchen sink and suddenly felt an unpleasant sensation in my groin.

Just a few days later, I was back at Memorial having surgery again, a second radical procedure on my left side. All my other leg and node surgeries had been on the right side. I left my practice. I retired. I thought I was going to die. I had metastatic melanoma. My marriage ended in 1985 and as a result, life actually became less stressful.

At least things were less stressful until it was discovered I had a cerebral metastasis on the right side of my brain. I was getting lost, acting strangely. The surgeon removed the cancer without doing further damage, but said, at a subsequent appointment, "There is no real treatment. Chemo will not be helpful for your type of cancer."

The year 1988 was a trying time. I developed a subdural hematoma and had a recurrence in the stomach that required surgical excision.

> **I sometimes wonder: When does a cancer victim make the joyous transition to becoming a survivor? For those who seek reassurance in statistics, the five-year mark bears a certain mystique.**

Whether justified or not, once having reached this arbitrary roadside marker these individuals and their families now breathe a huge sigh of relief. Right from the start, melanoma is different. Even when the magical fifth year has passed and despite sporadically reported instances of "spontaneous remissions," we never think of ourselves as "cured." Occasionally, even after a remission lasting as long as 20 years, this insidious disease has been known to return with grave consequences. On the sunniest of days a small, dark cloud still hovers on the horizon.

In December of 1988, at the suggestion of Dr. Abraham Mittelman, an immunologist, I embarked on an experimental monthly vaccination program. Its results would be uncertain. I had nothing to lose and side effects were supposedly nil.

Initially, my antibody response to the injections, based upon blood levels, was encouraging. I continued the program until December of 1991 and although I never suffered any side effects and was in remission, the program was eventually stopped due to the conclusion that it was considered ineffective. Only 10 to 15 percent of the patients had appeared to respond in any manner to the vaccinations.

Leg and Back Pain Dr. Steiner had suffered from leg pain, on and off, since the 1980s. This was considered to be a secondary issue in the wake of his cancer recurrences. During the early 1990s his pain continued in his legs and back, and was diagnosed as "neuropathic pain." On and off over several years, he had different scans and was prescribed different drugs and therapies to try and alleviate the symptoms. None of the drugs and other prescribed remedies relieved his symptoms for very long. The pain always returned.

Dr. Steiner was relieved that there was no evidence of further cancer recurrences, but his leg and back issues were chronic and at times severe. He continued to seek medical relief.

In 1996, Dr. Steiner had back surgery to try to relieve his chronic pain. Before long he began to experience pain in his right leg that awakened him from sleep. A short course of steroids failed to mitigate the problem.

More Cancer...Now in the Back

After an MRI, my doctor called, "I'm sorry to say that there's a small tumor mass in your lower back. It's intradural and appears to involve L5, the fifth lumbar nerve on the right. Obviously, we have to assume it's a recurrence of the melanoma."

I said, "I guess that would explain the pain I've been having all these months." He said, "Yes, it would." The tumor was removed with surgery the following week.

From time to time, Dr. Steiner continued to experience intermittent pain in his back. In March of 1997, he felt an unpleasant tingling pain underneath both buttocks. Over the next few days the sensation came and went. In an attempt to diagnose the problem, his neurosurgeon scheduled an MRI.

The doctor came in with the results. He said, "It's not good. Another intradural (tumor) recurrence not far from where the last one was. It looks to involve S1 on the right."

I had another surgery to remove this tumor. The next morning the surgeon came in and said, "I couldn't get it all out." The tumor had wrapped itself around the lower part of the spinal cord and if he attempted to remove it, I could have become a paraplegic without bladder or bowel control. The prognosis was bleak. This was an unsettling and scary time. My doctor prescribed chemotherapy pills, but the side effects proved to be much too challenging.

My physical strength and mental acuity were dwindling. My appetite declined until it vanished. I was miserable.

With the permission of my doctor I stopped taking the pills. A lumbar puncture had shown many cancer cells and elevated protein levels in my spinal fluid. The only option seemed to be to deliver chemo drugs into my spinal fluid, which might buy me two to three months.

You tend to go numb. You ask yourself, "What am I going to do?" There was little time to let this sink in. I tried chemo for a couple of weeks, but the side effects were so bad. Again, I quit the chemo.

Dr. George Wong, Traditional Chinese Medicine

I had investigated and called everyone in my Rolodex. There were not many, if any, options. The NIH (National Institute of Health) turned me down for any trials. Amidst the phone calls to medical people I knew, a doctor friend of mine who had been affiliated with the vaccination program I left, said, "I am going to suggest you call a fellow I know who is an expert in traditional Chinese medicine. Call Dr. George Wong."

I had nothing to lose; no one else had any ideas. I decided to see him. Dr. Wong had impressive credentials. He had a masters and Ph.D. from Harvard University.

When I met him he looked at me intently, performed a physical examination and said, "If you take the herbs that I'll have prepared for you, I think you can get over this." I asked, "Really?" He answered, "Really."

I started to take herbs. However, a couple of weeks later my oncologist called and told me about an expert in Texas who had good luck with my type of cancer. This doctor suggested injections of Interleukin-2 into my spinal fluid and to repeat these treatments, for an indeterminate period of time.

Dr. Wong forewarned me and said, "Interleukin-2 is very potent and can kill you, over time." I was not sure what to do.

Regardless, I tried the treatments and had them done in New York City. The side effects were very difficult. Each day was worse. I had pain and confusion. It was killing me, I felt wiped out. I bailed out after seven of nine scheduled treatments.

I went back to Dr. Wong and his Chinese herbs a few months later. His herbs are taken orally. After two to three weeks I was feeling much, much better.

I then decided to go to Europe to visit my mother for her birthday. I continued with the herbs, came back, had a couple more spinal taps and they were all clear!

I took the herbs for three years non-stop until the year 2000. I have never had any problem with melanoma since then. Dr. Wong's herbs dealt the melanoma cells a series of lethal blows and allowed my immune system to overcome the cancer.

In 2001, I developed prostate cancer. I did not have radiation or surgery to the dismay of my doctors, but took herbs specifically prescribed for my prostate cancer by Dr. Wong. Today, I continue to take these herbs for my prostate situation.

Transformation and Pearls of Wisdom

I think I was cancer prone, given the way I led my stressful, fast-paced life. I am sure it compromised my immune system over time.

The melanoma almost killed me, but in a sense it also saved me and led me to make major lifestyle changes. Today, I eat a much better diet. I have stayed with the herbs now for many years.

> **Regarding alternative medicine, obviously, there is a place for it. There are quacks, but there are all types of alternative care, much of which is effective.**

If anyone comes to me seeking my opinion about who has great knowledge and who can be very helpful, I say Dr. George Wong. George has had many great outcomes with many cancer patients over many years, including many advanced late-stage cancer situations. Unfortunately, the tradition of traditional Chinese medicine is being pushed off into the margins and trivialized. This is a real tragedy. Dr. George Wong is responsible for my being here today. He has unusual expertise and is phenomenal at what he does.

With his permission, I have included several quotes in this chapter from Dr. Nicholas V. Steiner's own book, *Unforeseen Consequences: A Physician's Personal Triumph Over Advanced Melanoma*.

MARK

Mark Olsztyn
Brain Cancer
Diagnosed in 1991

"You shouldn't waste your time talking to me. You should be getting your affairs in order and talking to God."
~Primary care physician's suggestion

His Early Years Although Mark's mom and dad divorced when he was only 7 years old, Mark estimates he had a fairly normal existence as a child. He continued to live with his mother and attended high school in Central Phoenix. He pointed out that he ate lots of junk food growing up and was exposed to a lot of second-hand smoke. His stepdad liked his Marlboros.

Meet Mark

After high school, I got a job in a tool-and-die factory where I was exposed to lots of different solvents. It was a time of aimless drifting. I worked as a busboy and at other odd jobs for about nine months before deciding to enroll at Phoenix College, a community college. Then, I transferred to Arizona State University and tried being a business major, but couldn't hack the accounting class.

I dropped out and went to work for my dad, who is a medical doctor, as a receptionist. It was a cushy job. I was living a hedonistic lifestyle geared towards the weekends, engaging in excessive partying and drinking with buddies, just wasting my time.

Something's Wrong

Fast forward to March of 1991. I was 26, living in Davis, California with my girlfriend of eight years, Belinda. On the night of March 1st, Belinda was awakened because she heard me making a hissing sound. I was shaking and writhing in my sleep. This wasn't just a bad dream; I was having a grand mal seizure.

Belinda called the paramedics who took me to a hospital. The CT scan indicated something, but the doctors weren't sure what it was. They called it "inconclusive." I would need an MRI. I called my dad and he arranged for me to come back to Phoenix for the scan. We needed to figure out what was going on.

On March 4th, I had an MRI. It indicated the presence of a brain tumor in my left frontal lobe. On April 4th, doctors at Barrows Neurological Institute in Phoenix resected a 2-centimeter Grade I Oligodendro Astrocytoma. It was explained that Grade I tumors require following up with MRIs every six months because there is a 50 percent chance of a recurrence. What I chose not to hear was that if it did come back, it would be much more malignant.

It was mind boggling to me. I simply couldn't grasp the reality of what was happening. With my head shorn and stapled, I entered into a denial phase that lasted almost exactly six years.

In August of 1991, I found a job doing news graphics at a TV station in Sacramento. No one at the station knew about my cancer, so I had to sneak away to get the MRIs and fret for days waiting for the results. Though the next two MRIs were clean, it was nonetheless horribly stressful for me.

When the evenings rolled around, I would get depressed. By barely dodging a bullet, I felt I had lost control of my destiny. I had the sense that God had issued me a warning to live life to its fullest and with purpose. I needed bigger challenges, so I applied to the Graphic Design program at Yale University and to my great joy received an acceptance letter. Belinda and I moved to New Haven. She worked as an intern in the hospital and I worked toward a master's degree.

Yale University

During my second year, Belinda became pregnant with our daughter. We hastily married and I graduated in 1995. Then we moved to Watertown, Massachusetts where I worked as a designer for a small but internationally renowned studio specializing in network packaging and branding. It was there that I met Marianna Gracey. She was my Project Manager and we became fast friends.

Belinda became pregnant with our son during this time. She and I were drifting apart, even before she got pregnant the second time. She relished her role as a mother, but had a hard time being a wife.

During the course of my friendship with Marianna, I shared my brain cancer story with her. At this time, both Lee Atwater, Chairman of the Republican National Committee, and the Oakland Raiders' Lyle Alzado had died of brain tumors. If these guys, with all of their connections couldn't be saved, well, I just couldn't face that. Who would I turn to if I had a recurrence?

Marianna knew someone who had breast cancer and told her friend about me, and the fact that I had not had any scans for many years. Her friend said, "If you really care about this guy, you will get in his face every day until he consents to getting scanned."

My Doctor

Because of Marianna's constant reminders, I went to see my primary care physician and explained to him, "The reason I have not followed up in getting scans over the years is the fear of what I may discover." He spoke directly to me, "Mark, look me in the eye; I would not lie to you. The fact that it has been six years and you are entirely asymptomatic tells me you will be fine. You need to get your head out of the sand."

Mark proceeded to get a brain scan despite being extremely stressed. On the day when Mark was going to get the results, St. Patrick's Day, 1997, he went home for lunch. Both kids happened to be sleeping.

He called his doctor's office and got him on the phone. The doctor said, "Mark, I have the results. Are you sitting down? They show a new tumor that is about five centimeters. I recommend we have it removed."

More Surgery

I was filled with dread and shock. It had come back after six years. One week later, I met with the doctor who was the Chief of Neurosurgery at a major Northeastern hospital.

Mark had surgery to remove the tumor, located in his left frontal lobe, using the latest surgical technique, a technique pioneered by this neurosurgeon. Regardless of the success of the surgery, the prognosis remained grim.

The neurosurgeon informed me that I had a Glioblastoma Multiforme, also known as a GBM. He explained that, unlike an Oligo, GBMs are the most lethal kind of brain tumor and that mine was considerably worse and more aggressive than my prior cancer. Surgery is just the first step. The doctor recommended I follow up with radiation and chemotherapy.

My heart sank to the floor. I felt hopeless. When I asked him how long I had to live, he responded, "It depends upon how you take to the treatment. No one can tell you that." In hindsight, those were healing words. As a lesson to all doctors who may read this, don't give a specific timeline of survival. I was so glad he did not give me a certain amount of months.

When a doctor gives you a timeline and says you only have three or six months to live, it can take away your hope and your ability to fight. On every statistical graph is the possibility of outliers. Why not me? This was dreadfully serious. All I wanted to know was that I had a chance.

The radiation treatment was terrifying. Fitted with a mesh mask, you have to remain very still as radioactive isotopes are beamed into your brain. I underwent 33 rounds of radiation—at the absolute maximum dosage—at this major hospital.

I wanted to see my doctor who had previously said, "You are going to be fine." I wanted him to tell me that again. I met with him and asked him, "I just have to know if anyone has ever survived this. Do I have a 10 percent chance?" He responded, "I wish I could say your chances are that good. You're wasting your time talking to me. You should be getting your affairs in order and talking to God."

His unsympathetic response really upset me, being so different from his prior reassuring words. For the first time, I really felt the gravity of my situation. I felt he was condemning me to death, and although I never felt more alone and despondent, I was determined to prove him wrong.

Next, I started but did not finish chemotherapy. I was supposed to go a full year of six rounds, but only went through four rounds. The chief of oncology was upset that I quit my chemo and issued a few cautionary tales of patients like me who suffered horribly after their cancer returned.

Poly MVA

I started taking a product called Poly MVA a few days after my surgery. My dad, a doctor involved in alternative medicine, sent me eight bottles. He had a colleague who had used it successfully. In 1997, there was very little information about it. I took Poly MVA simultaneously through my radiation and chemotherapy treatments, starting with a loading dose on April 4th, 1997. I have taken Poly MVA every day since then.

On the 11th anniversary of my surgery I visited my neurosurgeon and I could tell he was truly surprised I was still alive, but he was very happy to see me. I told him about Poly MVA, but like so many physicians, they won't consider it if it's not FDA approved.

I consider Poly MVA as the major force as to why I am alive and remain free of cancer today. In addition to Poly MVA, I now take vitamin D3, calcium,

CoQ10, iodine and green tea. I also meditate, take long walks and try to eliminate all stressors from my life.

During the initial stages of my recovery I took Chinese herbs and Essiac tea; I engaged in qui gong, visualization and acupuncture from time to time. I also took lots of other supplements that would support my immune system, if they were not contraindicative of any conventional treatments, and if they were reasonably priced.

Transformation and Pearls of Wisdom

I tell everyone who calls me for advice about cancer to get Dr. Bernie Siegel's wonderful book, *Love, Medicine and Miracles.*

**Do everything you can to improve your immune system.
Make sure your body is as healthy as you can make it.
Your immune system needs you now.**

One thing that really worked for me as far as the mind-body connection to wellness goes was listening nightly to Louise Hay's audio recording of "Self Healing: Creating your Health." It's available in many different formats these days.

Do not accept that your doctor or oncologist has the final word regarding how you will be affected by cancer.

**I am a bona fide, living survivor of a grim
prognosis. I am not a statistic.**

In 1997, I just wanted to talk to a single person who had survived 10 years beyond the diagnosis of Glioblastoma Multiforme. It's now 2016. In one more year I will have survived two decades.

I used to associate St. Patrick's Day with gloom. Now I celebrate it as the beginning of my lucky streak. A new chance at life!

SANDY

Sandy Yozipovic
Colon Cancer
Diagnosed in 2001

"Get your affairs in order, and go home and live your life."
~Two doctor's opinions at two major cancer centers

Her Early Years Sandy grew up in Saskatchewan, Canada. She was a farm girl, surrounded by lots of cattle, horses and pesticides. At the age of 21, Sandy was diagnosed with an autoimmune disease. She was partially paralyzed with a compromised immune system. The cold Canadian weather exacerbated her condition.

In 1997, at 35 years old, Sandy moved to Arizona. By 1999, she was experiencing extreme headaches. She was in so much pain for the next two years, on and off, Sandy sometimes found herself in a fetal position trying to will the pain away. This was a difficult conundrum, because despite her pain, she generally felt she was in good condition. She felt healthy. She competed in Tae Kwon Do tournaments and believed she ate a healthy diet.

During May of 2001, Sandy was having digestive problems. She had been passing blood for two to three months and finally decided to see a doctor at a major medical center in Arizona. The doctors at the center assured her that the pain and occasional bleeding were nothing serious, so she embarked on a trip to Canada to visit family.

There, Sandy became quite fatigued, needing two to three naps per day just to be able to function.

"Something's Wrong" On September 4th, 2001, Sandy went for a hike in beautiful Sedona, Arizona. As she walked down the trail, she experienced terrible stomach pain. The very next day she returned to the medical center in Phoenix where she underwent various tests and scans and was told on September 5th, 2001, that she had cancer.

Unbeknownst to Sandy at that time, her husband Mark was told that Sandy's situation was very serious. He did not want her to sink into a deep depression, give up, or become paralyzed with fear so he decided to hide the fact that she had advanced cancer. After a few days, Sandy was told the tumor was the size of her fist. She had surgery on September 11th, 2001.

Meet Sandy

The surgery lasted six hours—longer than anticipated. It confirmed my worst fears. I had an extremely serious colon cancer. Tumors were discovered in my rectum and through my intestinal wall. I was told I had Stage 4 cancer.

> **I was concerned; this could be it, but I had two young children and I wanted to be here for them. I thought it was my last Christmas.**

Sandy was not about to quit. She was young, and wanted to move forward and, as she said, "fight this thing."

Second Opinion

We met with Dr. Drew Collins of the Envita Clinic in Scottsdale for four hours talking about cancer, causes of cancer and ways to deal with it. He gave us hope that I could survive it. This was a great boost to my belief that this was not a death sentence.

I began a high-dose vitamin C therapy regimen, including changing my diet and adding specific health-building supplements, under the guidance of Dr. Collins. I wanted to strengthen my body, because I had decided I would probably get chemotherapy.

> Just two and a half weeks after surgery, Sandy and Mark boarded an airplane with just five passengers. It was eerily quiet; everyone was afraid to fly in the wake of 9/11. They were headed to a highly respected cancer center on the East Coast to get another opinion. They were on a fact-finding mission to learn whatever they could to maximize Sandy's odds of beating her cancer.

The doctor said, "So you had surgery four months ago?" Mark replied, "No, just about three weeks ago." The doctor was very surprised at my healthful appearance and the healing process of my scars in just three weeks. Of course, he did not know that I had recently begun a regimen of supplements and high-dose vitamin C therapy.

> Sandy proceeded to ask questions about alternative and unorthodox treatments, seeking the doctor's perspective about the therapies she had started as a result of her meeting with Dr. Collins at Envita. After Sandy's third question about the effects of dietary changes the doctor said, "Diet has nothing to do with cancer and dietary changes won't help you." He continued, "Other therapies are crazy. Anyone who recommends them is a quack. You have metastatic cancer!" The doctor was neither pleased nor amused with Sandy's desire to learn about integrative and alternative cancer-fighting options.
> Both the Arizona hospital and the East Coast cancer center recommended no more than 1,000 mg of vitamin C per day. Sandy was taking 65,000 mg intravenously per week!
> At the end of their consult, the doctor said he agreed with the Arizona doctors and said, "Go home and live your life."

Arizona Hospital

Back in Arizona, Sandy got started right away with a chemo regimen and radiation. Simultaneously, she followed an alternative path recommended by Envita, including supplemental IV vitamin C, as well as other supplements and treatments.

I asked my doctor at the Arizona hospital, "What vitamins would you recommend?" He did not respond with any recommendations. But fortunately, he was supportive of my desire to implement a variety of unorthodox treatments and therapies.

After four months, Sandy decided to stop her chemotherapy treatments.

The Arizona doctor told me, "Get your affairs in order."

Sandy's diet was now all organic; she abstained from dairy, "whites" (pasta, white rice, white flour, white potatoes), and caffeine. She became very diligent with her diet, eating lots of greens, and juicing daily to get nutrients and enzymes into her body.

I was off the charts regarding my white blood cells; they stuck together and created a perfect breeding ground for cancer. I needed to get rid of the acid in my body and alkalize it. Previously, I had been in the habit of drinking three cans of soda pop every day and protein shakes filled with sugar. I had thought I was eating a healthy diet.

Fighting peer pressure was a difficult grind.

Family and friends said, "Just listen to the Arizona doctors."
At times they created doubt about my choice, regarding an alternative path. I needed to do whatever I had to do, even though the odds were stacked against

me. You need to have a thick skin. I emailed friends instead of talking to them on the phone. I did not want to hear their negativity.

Your faith really comes into play; I am very spiritual. I read a book, *No Laughing Matter*, by Joseph Heller, about his cancer fight. It helped improve my attitude and got me through some tough times. You don't know if the decision you make will kill you or save your life. This was the most trying time. You have kids and a husband. Your family casts doubt on your sanity. I was scared. I wanted to stack the odds in my favor.

I questioned doctors, one by one, asking them, "If you were me, what would you do?"

Envita

From the first day I was released from the hospital after my surgery, I went to Envita every day for one year. Insurance did not pay for my treatments and therapies. It cost me over $40,000. My bill from the Arizona hospital, even with an 80/20 plan cost me $120,000. It is terrible how much cancer care costs and that integrative and alternative treatments are generally not covered by insurance. I was lucky that we could pay for my care.

Now, more than 15 years later, I go to Envita once per month for ozone therapy and high dose IV vitamin C treatments. We eat only organic food and pharmacy-grade supplements, as well. The type of supplements you take is critical; some have fillers and are not of the highest quality. I absolutely believe I would not be here if it were not for the doctors at Envita.

Transformation and Pearls of Wisdom

I now have so much knowledge compared to most people about integrative and alternative cancer care. I get calls from people all the time asking me, "What should I do?" When I was told I had cancer, I knew nothing.

When you are diagnosed with cancer, even Stage 4, it is not a death sentence. Educate yourself about nutrition; what to eat and what to avoid. Also remember: Attitude is critical.

ANTHONY

Anonymous Religious Leader
Prostate Cancer
Diagnosed in 1995

"I am so sorry."
~Doctor's comment, after cancer recurrence

His Early Years Anthony grew up in the Bronx, in New York City, in the 1940s and '50s. He was one of three brothers and experienced a happy upbringing. His parents were struggling, hard-working immigrants, constantly sacrificing for their children. Anthony lived in the city until he was 18 years old, where he finished high school, and then entered the seminary for the Catholic priesthood in New Jersey.

His journey took him to seminaries in New Jersey, Massachusetts, Ohio and New York. Anthony spent several years after ordination assigned to a parish in New York City. A true peripatetic lifestyle.

Then, the Superior overseeing his community wanted to send Anthony to Canada to develop an existing parish.

Meet Anthony

I was a bit depressed about it, being told to go to a different country to a new parish, but I went. That was over 30 years ago. First, I had my own new parish in this new area for about 10 years until 1993, then I joined the archdiocese and was sent to a parish for five years in an area one hour north of the city. Subsequently, I was assigned to another parish back in the metropolitan area. Now, I have been at my current church where I am today, with 3,000 families in our parish, since 2005.

Diagnosis

I asked Anthony if he had any warning signs or problems prior to his diagnosis.

Nothing specific. I was originally diagnosed when I was at the Canadian country parish north of the city. I had a nice country doctor whom I visited for an annual physical. He felt something suspicious during his digital exam and suggested I see a urologist.

The urologist said there was nothing to be concerned about, totally dismissing any concerns.

However, my country doctor wanted me to get a second opinion after he checked my PSA numbers again, informing me of an increase in the PSA.

Three months later, I went to a second urologist who performed a biopsy. I was very anxious. He said, "You have cancer." I was shocked. It was terrifying. I was in my 40s. I will never forget that day: December 8th, 1995. He recommended surgery. He said it was in the prostate gland and that, "We can get it all." At that time, I wanted surgery to get it out. If I could go back in time and change my mind, I would not have had the surgery.

A friend introduced me to Donald (Donnie) Yance of the Mederi Foundation prior to the surgery. Donnie is the preeminent expert in North America for botanical medicine pertaining to cancer treatment. He told me that cancer is systemic, not just localized. He said that cancer cells can be released into the body from a biopsy. At the time, I had a Gleason score of 8. He was not in favor of the surgery, however he was supportive of the decision I made.

After my surgery, according to the doctor, the pathology report indicated that the cancer was in the capsule and that they got it all. My PSA blood test indicated a reading of zero. Again, I was told that the cancer had not escaped.

Recurrence and Concerns

The doctors had been wrong. Contrary to my doctor's confidence after surgery, three years prior, the surgery did not get all of the cancer. The tumor was the size of a pea on the prostate bed. So, I went to a major hospital for cancer care in Canada around 1999, three years after my surgery. I had radiation treatments for a recurrence.

Donnie Yance guided me to certain products that would help support my immune system and help fight the cancer. Many of these products are specialized botanical supplements.

Discipline is really necessary when it comes to taking supplements and making serious changes.

I take them morning, noon and night. My supplement intake has increased over the years. Today, I take approximately 70 per day. Each supplement has a specific purpose, based on science. Donnie also offers strong advice as part of his protocol about lifestyle, foods to eat and avoid, exercise, and other health-inducing choices. He also wanted me to lose weight.

I had no side effects during my six weeks of daily radiation treatments. I believe Donnie's protocol was very helpful. When it was obvious that I had a recurrence, two different doctors said, "I am so sorry."

One was the doctor who had said, "We got it all." The other was a young radiologist at this esteemed hospital. I believe they were quite fatalistic in their comments. It was now assumed that I had cancer cells floating around my body.

After my radiation treatments, my PSA slowly increased over time, but was controlled by Donnie's protocol and constant tweaking, depending upon test results to monitor my prostate cancer. The PSA has gone up and down, but my work with Donnie has been constant.

I don't think I would be here if it wasn't for Donnie. The doctors at the hospital wanted to give me Lupron around 2010. Donnie suggested that I ask the doctors to give me Lupron, only intermittently. The Lupron would bring my PSA down to zero from 15, but then a couple years later it would escalate back up to 10 or 15. There are side effects to taking Lupron such as sleep disturbance and getting the sweats.

I have had anxiety about my cancer over the course of the past 21 years, but fortunately having Donnie in my life has made all the difference in the world. He is extremely knowledgeable and very supportive. Another priest, a friend of mine, had a similar prostate situation, and also took Lupron, but his situation was much worse. He did not have Donnie in his life.

Transformation and Pearls of Wisdom

Now, I have less fear about the word "cancer." It is ironic, that I have prostate cancer and that I am comforting people with it. Of course, they don't know I have it. Everybody is the same. There is the initial moment where everyone is frightened. However, I have come to the realization that cancer is something you can live with.

In 21 years, my personality has changed. I am not the same person I was. I am more patient with people. I see the big picture in life now, much more so than from many years ago.

The cancer experience puts things in perspective. I know that's a cliché, but you honestly do develop a different perspective. I would point people to the Mederi Foundation. Get Donnie Yance in your life. He is the "real thing" and cutting edge with his botanical oncology protocols. Unfortunately, too many people don't follow recommendations, but his have proven to work wonderfully well for me.

**The bottom line is, 'love, love, love.' Try to love people,
love life, feel the love of God. God is part of the picture.
I am thankful for my faith.**

Finally, the concept of hope is very important.

JOYCE

Joyce O'Brien
Breast Cancer
Diagnosed in 1998

"There is nothing we can do for you; Stage 4 is Stage 4."
~Doctor's opinion at a major cancer center

Her Early Years Joyce grew up in Queens, New York. Her mother was a retail department store employee and her dad was a New York City police officer. She went to a parochial high school, and grew up in a hard-working, caring, middle class family.

Joyce decided to get a jump-start on a career and made her way to Wall Street in 1984. At the age of 19, she found the corporate world to be both exciting and stressful. By the time she was 33 years old, she was a managing director responsible for 23 different hedge funds totaling $2.5 billion. She and her husband Kevin worked hard and played hard. In the midst of this fast-paced, non-stop financial world, Joyce dealt with chronic fatigue, sinus issues, daily headaches, irritable bowel syndrome, depression, and other health issues.

The unforeseeable trials and tribulations that would await the O'Brien family over the next few years would prove to become unrelenting, unimaginable.

Meet Joyce

Kevin had serious health issues prior to my cancer issues. I just assumed my health issues were normal. However, I was always tired.

One early morning in March of 1996, I headed off to work in Manhattan. My husband, then 31 years old, was still sleeping. Later that morning he called me and said, "I feel funny, I feel a bit numb." He was talking funny, as well. He had been out late with buddies the night before. I thought maybe he had a hangover. I called the doctor and described his symptoms. The doctor said, "Call the ambulance."

I left work and went home immediately. When I reached the house, the paramedics would not let me inside to see him. He was paralyzed. They thought it might be a stroke.

At the hospital, they said he had a brain hemorrhage. They didn't know if he would make it through the night. Friends and family gathered at the hospital. I stayed with him in intensive care all night. The doctor said, "I don't want to do brain surgery yet. I want to see if he can get any movement back and if the bleeding will stop." The doctor said my husband had experienced three strokes, and he told me, "We don't know if he will ever walk again."

> Shortly thereafter, Kevin did have brain surgery. Subsequently, he went through grueling physical therapy every day. Joyce worked shorter hours to spend more time helping out at home and nursing Kevin back to health. It was months before he could even move his big toe. Finally, over time, he got back 95 percent of the movement in his paralyzed leg.

In mid-1997, my company was being bought out. It was a most stressful, challenging time. I was also pregnant and the doctors thought my daughter had spina bifida. They wanted me to abort the child, but we chose not to. She came into the world just fine—no spina bifida.

Diagnosis: Breast Cancer Stage 2B

Kevin and Joyce had survived different episodes of serious stress. Two years had passed since Kevin's temporary paralysis and brain surgery. Eight months had passed since the birth of their beautiful, healthy daughter, coupled with Joyce's company having gone through a sale to another company. It was time to escape to a well-deserved vacation to the beautiful island of Jamaica.

We were in Jamaica. It was the first day of our vacation and I was taking a shower. I was thinking about a Barbara Walters special TV program I had seen concerning a woman named Erin Kramp.

Erin had a baby about the same age as mine. She had discovered a lump, breast cancer, which had metastasized. She was doing a series of videos for her daughter, so she would know her years later, because she knew she was going to die. Erin was on vacation when she discovered her lump. She was 33 years old at the time.

Suddenly, I felt a lump. I was 33 years old and I was also on vacation. I contacted my doctor from Jamaica. He said, "Come in when you get back, but I don't think it is anything serious." I went to my doctor upon returning and he sent me to another doctor who performed a biopsy.

It was cancer! I was freaked out! I was only 33 years old and had an 8-month-old daughter.

This was on May 7th, 1998. The cancer was diagnosed as extremely aggressive and in three out of four quadrants. Initially they said, "We don't think it's in the lymph nodes."

But they were wrong; it was.

Breast Cancer Surgery

My doctor said I needed surgery right away. I had a mastectomy at a major cancer hospital in New York City. The surgery took 10 hours and was filled with complications. I lost a lot of blood. In the recovery room I had convulsions and was numb. I had pain and a bad reaction to the anesthesia.

> **It was a horrific experience, minute by minute. I was**
> **praying and sometimes thinking, 'Maybe it would be**
> **easier to die.'**

After the surgery, which took place in July of 1998, I met with the oncologist. Her words incapacitated me. She said, "You can't have any more children, but you have an 85 percent chance of survival." I was blown away; I had wanted a big family. I went into a depression, constantly crying.

One month later I started chemotherapy. My episodes with chemo were on and off, increased and backed off, depending upon my immune system. I was in the ICU more than once since the chemo wreaked havoc with my blood cell counts. I lost my hair; I could not sleep in a bed for months, and had to sleep in a recliner. In fact, my blood cell counts were so far off, the doctors thought I had leukemia.

At this point, I was seeing many doctors.

Back to Work? Joyce was now recovering from surgery and her chemotherapy treatments. She had always worked hard in the fast-paced world of Wall Street, and wanted to get back to being productive again.

I wanted to go back to work. After being repeatedly assured that my job was safe, I was told that I no longer had a job and, therefore, lost my health insurance, my disability insurance and life insurance. It was devastating.

Now Kevin has Cancer

One year later, I was finally feeling somewhat better and we needed to get away. Kevin and I were about to depart for a vacation to Italy. There was a shrine that we wanted to visit to pray to a saint, whom we felt was helping us. Then just a few days before our trip, Kevin felt a lump in his groin. He wanted to delay going to the doctor until we returned, but I insisted that he go to the doctor, now.

He went to the doctor and had surgery to take out the lump. Two days later we went to Italy. While in Italy, from a payphone in a remote train station, our worst nightmares came true. We learned that Kevin had cancer, malignant melanoma.

When we returned home, we discovered that it was Stage 3b, maybe even Stage 4. The doctor said, "There are no good therapies for Kevin." This was in May of 1999, just one year after I was diagnosed with cancer.

I was now thinking, 'My daughter won't have any parents.'

The doctor told us Kevin had a 20 to 30 percent chance of survival. He said he could possibly get into a trial. We found a trial in New York with interferon and a vaccine. This was a very tough phase. I was still trying to get my strength back from my treatments and Kevin was having a tough time with his cancer. The trial was canceled shortly after Kevin started because too many people were dying.

Cancer Recurrence: Stage 4!

In October of 2000, life seemed to be improving. I finally found a new job and Kevin was doing OK. We decided to take a trip to Montauk, Long Island, to get away from the city for a few days. Something didn't feel right with me. We came back to our home and I went to the doctor. I had another lump in the same breast. It was a chest wall recurrence. It came through my skin and went into my neck. I also had spots on my lung and my liver.

After telling my oncologist and surgeon for over a year that I had a lump, and being told it was nothing to worry about, once it was confirmed to be cancer I was told, "It doesn't matter if we would have found it now or a year ago, we won't treat you. There is nothing we can do."

The doctor treated me like I was annoying him. I wanted to know that there was something else we could do. He said, "There is nothing we can do for you; Stage 4 is Stage 4."

Joyce had been through so much. Her doctor gave her no hope and told her to get her affairs in order. She could not imagine that this was the end, and that her daughter would grow up without parents. Although she was desperate and in despair, there was still an underlying desire burning deep inside her, that she would not be beaten.

I visited with a woman who had made my dress suits. She suggested I call someone whom she said might be helpful. I was very skeptical, but made an appointment. I had nothing to lose. But I wondered:

How could alternative stuff possibly be as effective as conventional medicine? I had never even been in a health food store before being diagnosed with cancer, but I needed to live and that meant trying anything.

This "someone" was not a doctor, but an alternative practitioner. This person looked at my blood and said it did not look healthy. He looked into my mouth and said I had mercury poisoning. He said, "I think I can help you."

I had lived on sugar, pasta and pizza. I was encouraged by this practitioner to radically change my diet to mainly raw greens and shots of wheat grass daily. The wheat grass is great for detoxification. Also, I was directed to take certain supplements and homeopathic remedies. I stayed loyal to the green diet and other supplements and remedies. I was feeling much better after three weeks. After four weeks I felt great for the first time in my life!

Then, I went to Kevin's oncologist. Despite the dire prognosis of my oncologist, his oncologist said we could try radiation and low dose chemotherapy, and continue with Herceptin.

I had the alternative practitioner look at my blood again after four more weeks, and it looked great. I then decided to start back with conventional radiation and low dose chemo for eight weeks. I felt terrible, again. All the old symptoms started to come back.

I continued with the holistic path, simultaneously with the conventional treatments. Regarding the issue of taking supplements while on chemo, the doctor said, "I don't want to know if you are going to do supplements and homeopathic treatments, simultaneously. I don't want to know anything about it." But, she did not tell me to stop, because it was Stage 4 and she had seen other people who had great results using supplements and other alternative treatments, at the same time as radiation or chemo. Her nurse's daughter had obtained wonderful results from alternative therapies with another health issue, so she was more open to other approaches.

Switzerland Cancer Clinic

Joyce was on an aggressive mission to do everything she could to beat her cancer with whatever means possible. The alternative practitioner in New York spoke of a cutting-edge cancer clinic in Switzerland called Paracelsus. He felt this clinic could do wonders for Joyce's precarious situation and hopefully tip the odds in her favor.

It was a godsend for me to be at this clinic, in the German area of Switzerland.

**My family thought I was nuts to go to Switzerland,
but they remained supportive.**

Kevin brought me there for three weeks in February of 2001. The clinic used a multi-faceted approach. The treatments included IV therapies, homeopathic therapies, ozone, hyperthermia, vitamin C, colonics, live blood analysis, Iscador, psychological work and energy work.

Additionally, I was put on a strict dietary regimen: lots of special supplements and other treatments. The conventional doctors back in the States saw progress through their scans. I went back to Switzerland again in July of 2001 for another two weeks of intensive therapies and treatments; then again in January of 2002 to an affiliated clinic for two more weeks. Then, more visits two years later and then again, two years after that.

The conventional doctors said the cancer was gone approximately nine months after my first visit to the clinic in Switzerland. They were startled, acknowledging that the scans could not detect any cancer. The holistic doctors disagreed and said, "You are not in the clear." They did not show the same confidence until I was 18 months out from my first treatments in Switzerland.

Through her intensive diet and lifestyle changes, combined with repeated, customized treatments and therapies received in Switzerland, Joyce's body and immune system became strengthened and the cancer weakened. She has remained vigilant and continues to maintain an extraordinarily healthy lifestyle so the cancer does not rear its ugly head once again. She monitors her health regularly, and tweaks her regimen on an ongoing basis to ensure that she stays healthy.

Another clinic she visited in the U.S. was the Hippocrates Clinic in Florida. At Hippocrates, Joyce said, "I did infrared saunas, wheat grass implants (enemas), nutritional regimens, supplementation and other healing treatments." Joyce ultimately studied many of these modalities that she used to heal herself, so that she could help others heal as well.

Miracle?

Approximately five years after Joyce was declared cancer free, she met with a new oncologist. The oncologist looked at Joyce's records and said, "There must be a mistake. Your records say you have aggressive Stage 4 cancer, but there is no sign of it in any of your test results."

Joyce responded, "No, I am cancer free now for five years." The doctor continued and said, "Something is wrong or this is a miracle." Joyce responded again, "No, it is not a miracle. Perhaps it is a miracle that I found the right path, but it is based on science and rational medical reasons."

Transformation and Pearls of Wisdom

The most important thing was the homeopath, the alternative practitioner who gave me hope and said, "I think I can help you." This is a huge factor towards enhancing survival. Having hope is huge. It disturbs me when doctors give you time frames.

When someone says, "You are cancer free," that does not mean you stop doing what you are doing. You must continue doing all kinds of healing treatments and therapies.

You must get to the root causes of why you got cancer. You must reduce stress in your life. You must cut out all sugar and simple carbohydrates. Go raw green for the initial period of time. You also need to detox, slowly. You should get tested for heavy metals and food intolerances that suppress the immune system, as well. You should eliminate dairy from your foods.

In order to heal you must address the physical, environmental, mindset, emotional and spiritual issues that lead to cancer and remove those causes so the body can build itself back up again and heal.

I do not recognize the person I was before. I don't know that person. We are meant to feel fantastic, to get to root causes and allow ourselves to heal.

Both Kevin and I have radically changed our lifestyles and we are both very healthy and passionate about living life. I am happier now than I have ever been!

ANNIE

Annie Brandt
Breast Cancer
Diagnosed in 2001

*"If you don't do a double mastectomy, chemo and radiation,
you will probably die within three to six months."*
~Doctor's opinion

Her Early Years Annie was born in Milwaukee, Wisconsin, one of four siblings. Her father was a salesman and her mother was a housewife. Her father often came home from work tired, irritated, and was quick to anger. When she was about 8, her mother became an alcoholic. Annie's home life was, in her words, "a bit dark." She felt alone, somewhat inferior and unworthy in her own house, feeling she was not good enough. Her parents seemed to have special feelings toward her twin siblings and brother, but not towards Annie.

Meet Annie

I was a people pleaser, trying to always make things right. I had what is called a typical cancer personality. I was "Little Miss Fix-It." I put everyone else first and tried to make everyone else happy. It was a stressful childhood. The twins were super achievers. Academically, I got very good grades, but not great. I could not compete with the twins.

When I was 14 years old, the family moved to St. Louis. It was culture shock to me. I went from a small school to a large school, from the country to the busy suburbs. I was shy and awkward, and felt inadequate. I constantly carried and buried a lot of stress, and did not express my feelings.

After studying business and marketing in college I went to work with Anheuser Busch as a secretary, the only way I could get in. I worked very hard and was promoted within one year to market research specialist, where I handled important, special projects for upper management. It was in this role where I was exposed to computers. Soon thereafter a computer company recruited me as a systems engineer, and I began my career in computers.

In 1985, I moved to San Antonio, Texas. I developed allergies to "everything that grows," according to the doctor. In 1987, I also developed intestinal allergies to hormones and antibiotics in beef. I now know that the onset of allergies is a sign that your immune system cannot keep up with what is bombarding it.

Not Feeling Great

In 1992, I was a corporate information networking consultant, one of very few people anywhere at that time who performed this function. I was working 60 to 80 hours per week supporting Fortune 100 companies, and I was at the top of my professional path.

But then I started to get sick. First I got what I thought was the flu, but it would not go away. After six months and numerous tests, I was diagnosed with chronic fatigue immune dysfunction syndrome, also known as CFIDS. I thought it was nothing and that I could shake it, but it was very debilitating and lingered on. The doctors said, "We don't really know what to do about CFIDS, and we don't have anything to give you other than medication for the side effects."

I started doing my own research with the goal of healing myself.

In 1992 I watched a Bill Moyers program on public television, "Healing and the Mind." It gave me insight and hope that I might be able to cure my CFIDS. I tried different kinds of mind-body treatments.

Next, I found a diet that connected yeast with CFIDS, so I investigated dietary changes to heal. I was also taking wild blue green algae supplements to detox and nourish at the cellular level and was now feeling a little better.

In 1994, on a very memorable day, I became extremely dizzy. I could not stand up and began vomiting, which continued for 13 days straight. I went to the hospital and was diagnosed with Multiple Sclerosis (MS).

I then went to Duke University to confirm the diagnosis and was told I had both CFIDS (I knew that) and MS. I was so despondent, I felt somewhat suicidal about my situation.

Shortly thereafter, my mother's friend from church came over and brought me a book about diet and MS. The book said, "MS patients should avoid dairy and yeast." When visiting, she told us about a gentleman from Florida who owned a health food store who had MS, and had developed a supplement program to go along with the MS diet. On his program and the diet, he had started out in a wheelchair, then graduated to a walker, then a cane, and is now playing tennis. This opened my mind to diet and supplements for MS that might cleanse and strengthen my body.

Stress and More Problems The next five years brought about more stress and health problems for Annie.

In 1995, my doctors diagnosed me with mitral valve prolapse, a heart problem. Ugh, more issues on top of the CFIDS and MS challenges. In 1996, I met my future husband. In 1997, we moved to Austin, Texas to start a green design and build company.

That same year, I developed chemical sensitivity problems and my immune system became overwhelmed again. I bought an air purifier and brought plants into the house, which helped my problems immensely. This is when I learned that environmental issues are another key to causing and healing chronic disease.

In 1998, my future husband and I bought a lot in Austin and made plans to build four green houses on the lot. Then in 1999, I got married and was shocked one week later when I was contacted by the IRS. I learned that my husband owed back taxes of $165,000 that I was now also responsible for. I was blown away because he had never told me about this debt. Around the same time, several customers also sued the company. Needless to say, this was all a huge shock, especially to a newlywed who still had her rose-colored glasses on! This all brought about a great deal more stress.

Diagnosis

The stress of the prior years had taken a toll on me, and it was about to manifest itself in a physical form. On the 4th of July 2001, I was taking a shower and found a lump under my left arm. It was literally not there the day before.

I made an appointment to see my gynecologist who sent me for a mammogram, but nothing showed up. Then, I had an ultrasound. The doctor said the results looked odd. Then, I was shuffled off to a surgical oncologist who said, "Let's be safe and not sorry." She biopsied the swollen lymph node on July 13, 2001; it was Friday the 13th.

I was in the recovery room, still pretty groggy, and the doctor came in and said, "Sorry, but you have cancer and it is at least Stage 2, because it is in the lymph system."

**My world stopped. I was thinking, 'Oh my God,
I have cancer and I am going to die.'**

The doctor proceeded to tell me, "I have you booked for a double mastectomy next Tuesday" (four days later) and then she just walked out. She had no bedside manner. A good friend brought me to this appointment. She was talking to me; I could see her lips move, but I could not hear a word she was saying. All I could think was, "I am going to die, I am going to die, I am going to die...."

That night, I went home and cried and cried. It was 2:00 a.m. My husband came out of the bedroom and said, "You are keeping me awake; please stop it."

I was so tired of all the health challenges and the stress, and said to myself, "God, please take me now," but I also heard a voice say, "I love you. I won't let anything happen to you."

The voice was so real that I looked around, thinking someone had broken into the house. Then I realized, I was hearing the voice of God. I know most people would think I was crazy, but it was that real. And suddenly, it all made sense to me. I understood that I had nothing to worry about; if I died, I was going to God and if I lived, I would have a story that would help others.

I sat up in the recliner, went to the bedroom, got on the Internet and began to research everything I could think of to help me deal with the cancer. I found out that surgery weakens the body and the immune system.

When I researched conventional chemo and radiation, I found out that they did a lot of detrimental things. They can: kill the P53 tumor-suppressor gene, the very gene you need to fight cancer; distort the DNA of your healthy cells making them pre-cancerous; weaken the immune system; damage the vital body organs; cause cancer to build up immunities against the chemo and radiation; and, have many violent side effects, severely impacting quality of life.

On Monday, at my pre-op session, I talked to my doctor and asked her a lot of tough questions about the results of my research on surgery, chemo, and radiation side effects. She acknowledged that all of my points were true.

I told her I did not want to follow her suggestion of a double mastectomy, chemo, and radiation.

You Will Probably Die Within Three to Six Months

My surgical oncologist was quite upset with my decision. She said, "If you don't do this you will probably die." I told her that, if I was going to die, I was going with as many of my original body parts and as much dignity and quality of life as possible.

As I searched for better options and answers, I found a doctor in Houston, Texas. He did scans, found more lesions in my lungs and in my brain. I told him I wanted to do as much natural and non-invasive things to my body as possible. He said, "Hurry and get your affairs in order." He held out little hope for me. It is hard to stay positive with that kind of message.

I went to a different oncologist who also suggested the "standard of care" trio of surgery, chemotherapy, and radiation. I challenged him with my research and he agreed that it was all true. So I said, "Well, why would I want to do that?" And he said, "If you don't, you will probably die within three to six months."

I told him that God was the only one who knew when I was going to go, and that everyone else just had an opinion. I also told him that I didn't want to do surgery, chemo, and radiation. The doctor became livid and yelled at me saying that I was going to die if I didn't do what he told me to do. I told him, "I am firing you." He said, "You can't fire me." I said, "Watch me!" I told the HMO I wanted a different doctor. After a few conversations, they complied.

I did start a program with the Houston doctor's recommendation to take sodium phenylbutyrate, but I had a toxic reaction to it. In my continuing research, I found a cleanse at the Optimum Health Institute in Texas which provides patients with a total organic raw vegan diet, heavy juicing, wheatgrass, a whole body cleanse, enemas, colonics, exercise, yoga, food classes and other natural remedies.

I stayed at this clinic for seven weeks, and felt much better. I learned that the order of what you eat is very important. Juices digest most quickly, then fruits, then vegetables. Raw digests first, then cooked.

After the fruits and vegetables, the order of digestion is: starchy vegetables, grains, starches, fish, chicken, pork, beef. If you eat meat, make it organic meat, but eat it last, because it progresses through the digestive system slower than anything else. So if you eat the meat first, then the potato, then the vegetables, the potato and vegetables have to wait for the meat to digest before it goes through your intestinal tract. This means you have food just sitting around in your digestive tract.

I stayed raw organic vegan for seven and a half months, and then gradually added cooked foods and a little organic meat back into my diet. I felt very good and the scans were showing that the tumors were generally staying the same, but I also had some shrinkage.

Still, people were pushing me to have the double mastectomy, chemo and radiation. I rejected their advice; it was tough. I lost a few friends in the process, but I felt it was important, as the medical profession states, "First do no harm."

In 2002, a year after I was told I would live three to six months, I found more lumps under both arms.

My conventional doctor again tried to talk me into a double mastectomy, chemo and radiation. I went back to the Internet and library to do more research.

Insulin Potentiation Therapy

I continued trying to find good options. One day, I found something called Insulin Potentiation Therapy (IPT). I read of someone who had end-stage breast cancer who implemented IPT and survived. When I could not find any IPT doctors in the U.S. (by the way, that has all changed since the advent of Best Answer for Cancer Foundation), I called Dr. Donato Perez Garcia in Mexico, the grandson of the inventor, and sent him my records. He said, "I won't make you promises, but I think I can help you." He was the first doctor who said he could help. Kind, welcoming words.

I flew to San Diego, took a trolley to the border, then took a taxi to Dr. Donato's clinic. He explained the treatment plan, and we set up an appointment. The next day, I went in fasting, and he hooked me up to an IV after checking my weight and vitals. He then injected a small amount of insulin into an IV, based on my body weight. I sat there with my book, and after about 20-25 minutes, the doctor checked my pulse and asked, "How are your eyes?"

My eyesight was a little blurry, my pulse was elevated, and I was flushed. He said I was in a slightly hypoglycemic state, which was what he called the "therapeutic moment." This is the moment that the cancer cells are heavily involved but the healthy cells are not. He was now ready to deliver the chemo, 10 percent of the regular dose, into the IV.

He also delivered a liver support injection, anti-inflammatories, antibacterials, antivirals, and antifungals into the IV. The very last thing was glucose; the glucose serves to help seal the chemo into the cancer cells and brings you out of a hypoglycemic state that completes the treatment.

The procedure took 45 minutes to an hour. I flew home the next day, and I felt great. I had energy. I did this treatment twice per week for one month, then once per week for six weeks. He kept backing off the frequency of the treatments as the cancer responded. It is not like conventional, where you do a round of chemo and then have to rest the body because you are so sick. The therapy was easy for me, and I never had any side effects.

By March of 2003, my tumors were all gone, according to a PET scan done by my regular oncologist. I was in remission.

Personally, I don't believe in the concept 'cancer free,' but I believe you can be 'cancer quiet' or 'cancer clear.'

Then, I was put on maintenance for IPT—approximately once every three months, then once every six months for a year, then once per year. Now, I also go to a doctor in the Dallas area, Dr. Constantine Kotsanis, who gives me IPT once per year as well as integrative treatments to support my immune system.

In 2004, I was diagnosed with type 2 diabetes. My marriage was very stressful and my husband had been abusive towards me for years. One night, he became physically abusive. The abuse was traumatic, too much to take. I left him.

Non-Profit Foundation

In August of 2003, I was thinking of starting a non-profit foundation related to IPT for cancer, and I was going to call it Best Answer for Cancer. Dr. Donato was excited about it, but I ran out of money while I was setting it up.

In 2004, Dr. Donato called and told me about a woman named Rachel Best who also wanted to start a non-profit regarding IPT. Her last name, Best, and my idea for the name were too serendipitous to ignore. Rachel and I started our foundation shortly thereafter, named The Elka Best Foundation, after Rachel's mother who died of cancer.

In January of 2005, Rachel went to the hospital to get a tumor debulked, but then became very sick with an infection. The hospital stabilized her and sent her home, but she went back to the hospital shortly thereafter.

After two months of trying to treat the infection, Rachel died. The doctors think she died of an aggressive, lethal infection, MRSA. It was a trying time. I had two paid consultants but only about $46 in the foundation's bank account. I called the two consultants, offered them directorships in the foundation in exchange for them to help me for free. They agreed. I immediately recruited three IPT physicians as board members and formed the organization as a 501(c)3 nonprofit. I changed the name to "Best Answer for Cancer."

Current Times

Today, I have been cancer clear for 15 years. I still get IPT once per year and do other integrative therapies to heal and nourish the body such as Ultraviolet Blood Irradiation (UBI), ozone, high-dose vitamin C, and enzymes. I still practice the whole-being healing that I developed through all of my other illnesses.

Cancer builds up an immunity to treatments, so it is important to switch things around. Keep it at bay with different patterns, different supplements, different treatments. I walk, do yoga, colonics, visualization and prayer. I also take lots of supplements, drink lots of Essiac tea and sometimes take Chinese herbs.

Transformation and Pearls of Wisdom

My quality of life is excellent. I love life, I love what I do, and when I put my head on the pillow at night, or at the end of my life, I know I will have done good things and that I have helped people.

Cancer was probably the best thing that ever happened to me. It awakened me to living life with intention, and with grace. Cancer forced me to go back and look carefully at my life.

I tell patients: If you have cancer, the first and most important thing is to do your research. You have time. The cancer has been growing for a long time;

you have a week or two to get the facts. Then, put plans into place to engage in treatments and therapies that will help, and filter out the "noise" of misinformation, the naysayers, and well-meaning yet ignorant people. Understand that knowledge is power, and attitude is everything. Get rid of everything negative and pick good tools to help your mind.

And remember, "God is large and in charge."

You need to address the whole being with many tools, some of which are: self-hypnosis, meditation, visualization, exercise, nutrition, raw veggies, light organic meats, colonics, supplementation, spirituality, prayer, good rest, liver support, laughter, classical music, positive thoughts (negative thoughts suppress the immune system), all of these things. You do whatever you need to do.

With my prior illnesses, I asked, "Why me?" I no longer feel that I am a victim. It is fine, it is all good. I have had a fantastic experience, admittedly amidst some trauma, but overall it has been an incredible experience.

Get involved in life. Get involved with your treatment plan. What will you do outside of what the doctor wants you to do? What will you do to be happy?

Remember to put yourself first. It's like they tell you on the airplane, "Put the oxygen mask on yourself first and then worry about others around you." Because if you die, how can you help anyone?

Listen to your body, live now, live today. Every day is the first day of the rest of your life. Decide how you are going to live life and get on with it.

DAVID

David Hanbidge
Lung Cancer
Diagnosed in 1999

"Get your affairs in order."
~American Cancer Society employee, Long Beach, CA

His Early Years David, an only child, was born in February, 1945, in Hamilton, Canada. His mother was a schoolteacher and his father a tool maker who ran a Best Foods plant. The family moved to Cleveland, Ohio when David was 8 years old where his father took a job with Ford Motor Company. This was a difficult time for David as his mother and father had a troubled, dysfunctional relationship.

Meet David

My mom had mental problems. She could function, but was somewhat delusional and extremely religious. She would do irrational things, claiming Jesus told her to do them. When I was 13 years old, my mother ran off with someone she met at church. That same year she was put in a mental institution in Douglas, Arizona.

My dad had custody of me. We moved a lot, from Ohio to Phoenix, to Bisbee, Arizona, and back to Ohio in 1959. My mother died of cancer in the mental institution. Dad remarried and I went to work in a restaurant.

In September, 1969, David was 24 years old. He moved to Hollywood, California and was fortunate to land a good job with a bank. He worked hard, climbed the corporate ladder and became a vice president in 1973. He subsequently left the bank in 1984 to start his own business, a used car dealership in Rosemead, California. Business was steady, David was making good money, and he developed a solid, reputable company.

Warning Signs

In August of 1998, I was on vacation in Italy. I experienced chest congestion and low energy. I coughed whenever I tried to take a deep breath. I had been a smoker since I was around 10 years old. Upon returning in the States I went to the doctor who said it must be allergies.

In January of 1999, my dad got lung cancer and died just a few months later, in April. He had also been a smoker.

My low energy, coughing and the heaviness in my chest persisted, so in the summer of 1999 I had a chest x-ray. The doctor said I had pneumonia, but I also had a normal white blood cell count.

Despite the doctor's diagnosis, David was troubled. How could he have pneumonia and a normal white blood cell count? He decided to investigate his condition further, especially since he was now coughing up traces of blood.

He saw Dr. Cameron Dick, a pulmonary specialist, in August 1999, who performed a bronchoscopy procedure, chest x-ray and a CT scan. The bronchoscopy was revealing, where the other scans were not determinative of David's condition. His problem was hidden in the lower lobe of the left lung, behind his heart, and was difficult to see with the scans. During the procedure, David was coughing up blood. The resulting diagnosis was shocking.

Dr. Dick said, "This is not good; this is serious." I will never forget the day when Dr. Dick took my wife and me to a small back office and told us the horrible news. I had the very worst kind of lung cancer, primary small cell lung cancer.

I remember Dr. Dick had tears in his eyes when he told us the news. He told us the outlook of surviving this kind of cancer was very bleak. We were stunned. Nothing prepares you to get this kind of death sentence.

Dr. Dick said, "If it were me or my father, there is only one man I would see. I used to ridicule his work, but he has survivors that no one else has. His results speak for themselves." Dr. Dick explained that this doctor was considered a bit of a renegade, that he used non-traditional approaches and sometimes, unconventional chemotherapy medicines. Despite his unorthodox approach, the news of his results was spreading and this doctor's reputation was growing.

Despite Dr. Dick's hope that this oncologist might help me, I still had small cell lung cancer, confirmed by the biopsy. The prognosis was truly bleak. I did not want to die.

I got on the computer and looked for survivors. I could not find a survivor of small cell lung cancer lasting more than six months. I was so shaken, scared to death. Although my wife was also shaken, she would not let me quit. She would not let me go down without a fight.

New Hope: Robert Nagourney, M.D.

Dr. Dick picked up the phone and called Dr. Robert Nagourney. David and his wife were too shaken, too shocked to make such a call. Fortunately, Dr. Dick persuaded Dr. Nagourney to see David during the next few days, despite Dr. Nagourney's heavy patient demands.

A few days later, I was sitting in Dr. Nagourney's office. Dr. Nagourney said, "Statistically, people with your type of cancer have a 5 to 10 percent chance of survival of five years."

That same week, I went over to the American Cancer Society in Long Beach, California where an employee of the Society said, "Get your affairs in order. Lung cancer is not curable."

Dr. Nagourney approached chemotherapy differently from most doctors in the U.S. Before beginning his atypical chemotherapeutic regimen, David had surgery to remove the lower left lobe of his left lung. Dr. Nagourney wanted to obtain a tissue sample of the cancer from David's lower left lobe for analysis in his lab. The sample was excised during the surgery.

I was looking for hope from Dr. Nagourney, but he was quite conservative when commenting about my prognosis.

Unique Chemosensitivity Test

Dr. Nagourney is one of only two doctors in the U.S. who test cancer cells and tissue samples of the actual patient, in a very specific and unique manner. Many doctors and cancer centers claim to do chemosensitivity tests; however, the methodology of these doctors varies widely from the lab tests done at Dr. Nagourney's lab.

Many doctors claim that Dr. Nagourney's unique test does not work, that it is unproven, but there are many other doctors and patients throughout the nation who disagree and state that his patients' outcomes are superior compared with conventional outcomes.

David's cancer tissue was tested against many different combinations of chemotherapy drugs to ascertain which combination produced the best results. The goal was to evaluate sensitivity and responsiveness of the cancer to the drugs. Dr. Nagourney does not make decisions about using drugs based specifically on large randomized trials generated from thousands of "other people." Instead, he uses singular chemo drugs or combinations that are shown to be effective for his specific patients, from his own lab work. The results of Dr. Nagourney's laboratory work engender a personalized/customized chemotherapeutic drug or combination of drugs, for each individual. He performs "the test" not only for his patients, but for patients nationwide and worldwide, when requested by their doctors.

It makes sense that there is no "one size fits all" approach to cancer treatment. The success lies in matching the most formidable chemo drug(s) against a particular, specific cancer tissue.

That fact was undeniably proven when it was determined that the application of chemotherapy drugs traditionally used to fight breast and brain cancers, were among the best weapons to fight my specific lung cancer. The test shows what is best, as opposed to an off-the-shelf regimen.

Dr. Nagourney had mentioned a recent study in England that produced favorable numbers. Unlike many oncologists, he stays on top of the latest studies. He followed this protocol in his approach with me, twice per day, which included radiation and the chemo shown to be effective for me. One week of treatment, then three weeks off, then another week on and three weeks off, continuously.

I did have some side effects and significant nausea from the chemo, but I only threw up once. The radiation did, however, make me weak. At the end of 11 months, Dr. Nagourney said, "I have given you all the chemo I can give you, but I can't find any signs of the cancer. If it comes back, it will probably come back in the brain."

Then, two months later, because of Dr. Nagourney's concerns about the severity of my small cell lung cancer and the real possibility of a recurrence, especially in the brain, he wanted to embark on more treatments, despite the fact that he was concerned about more chemo. His concerns about the cancer spreading to my brain were greater than his concerns about giving me more chemo.

Dr. Nagourney said there is one chemotherapy drug that pierces the blood-brain barrier. He said, "This has never been done, but I am suggesting that we do one month of brain radiation, coupled with this chemo drug."

I agreed. I trusted Dr. Nagourney and wanted to do everything I could to prevent any kind of a recurrence. He wanted to take action to eradicate any cancer that might be lurking in my brain.

Mind-Body Walks

I am not a religious person or a member of any organized religion, but I prayed every day, especially when I walked. Every day after getting chemo treatments, I walked two hours at a local nature preserve and visualized that the chemo was attacking and defeating my cancer. I tried to stay positive about my chances of winning this war.

You must continually fight the cancer with your mind. I can't say scientifically that it helped, but I know it didn't hurt and I believe my walks, coupled with my prayer and visualization, were helpful in my efforts to beat my cancer.

Then, I met someone with small cell lung cancer while doing chemo in 2000. He had survived over 15 years. This gave me great hope, to actually meet someone who had great success. This gave me a real boost!

> Besides putting his dire prognosis in Dr. Nagourney's hands, and the doctor's unique protocol and chemo drugs that were derived from his novel lab work, David did not implement any other extraordinary strategies. He did, however, cut down on red meat consumption, and took the supplements CoQ10 and L-carnitine, as well. Occasionally, he took turmeric which has a powerful active agent known as curcumin. Also, since his diagnosis, David has never picked up a cigarette.

Transformation and Pearls of Wisdom

I look at things differently now. If I don't enjoy what I am doing, I don't do it for long. The most precious thing is not money, not a diamond, not a big house; it is health and time. Don't waste time.

If someone wants to know what to do if they get cancer, I have two words for them: Rational Therapeutics (the name of Dr. Nagourney's practice and laboratory). Insist that your oncologist work with Rational Therapeutics.

Do the test. I am here today because of Dr. Nagourney.

I just see a regular doctor now, once per year, and have seen him for the past seven years for chest x-rays and a physical.

**If you can do something for other people, it is helpful
to you. Be a giving person. Negativity can kill you.
Maintain a positive attitude, always.**

I feel great now! I am the luckiest man on earth!

JOSHUA

Joshua Pock
Brain Cancer
Diagnosed in 2005

"Joshua has about 18 months to live."
~ER doctor, talking to Joshua's father

His Early Years Joshua grew up in Sacramento, California and the Lake Tahoe area. His parents, as he put it, were "hippies." His father played guitar in an opening act for the Grateful Dead; however, his father is now a very successful owner of a software company.

In his younger years, Joshua enjoyed the great outdoors, specifically the forest and backpacking. Despite the outward appearance of being a typical adolescent, he was always self-conscious, a bit depressed and constantly trying to find himself. In his early high school years, Joshua was diagnosed as bipolar.

Meet Joshua

My doctor prescribed lithium for me to deal with my bipolar issues. It just numbed me. It flattened my personality.

After high school, Joshua went to junior college and later received a degree in forest conservation (Forestry) at Humboldt State University in 1999. After graduation, he became involved in fire-fighting and tree marking work in Northern California, measuring trees and taking stock of the forest for loggers.

Warning Signs

I started slowing down, I couldn't keep up with the daily workload. As a result, my pay was reduced. I began suffering from frequent headaches around 2004 and because I could not handle my workload well, I lost my job in forestry. I soon realized that forestry was not for me anymore. In hindsight, I attribute my inability to work in a focused manner to my brain tumor.

My wife and I moved back to Rocklin, California, where I went to work for my father. He hired me to work in quality assurance, testing software for his software development company.

I started having more headaches at work and went to appointments with different doctors. Some said the headaches might exist because I was staring at a computer monitor all day. I also had floaters in my eyes, along with the continual migraines, including a weird metallic taste that persisted in my mouth. I had also passed out twice, once at work and once in the shower for no reason that I could understand, waking up with the left side of my body totally numb. No one could figure it out. I maxed out on Advil and Excedrin and slept a lot trying to escape my headaches. I felt something was wrong.

You Have Brain Cancer

In April of 2005, I attended a Christian men's conference with my father at Lake Tahoe. I told him about my symptoms and he proceeded to talk to an ER doctor at the conference about my issues. The ER doctor said, "Come to my hospital in Truckee for a brain scan." We did, and the scan indicated that I might have brain cancer. On April 22, 2005, I had a biopsy and it was confirmed: I had a malignant brain tumor. The doctor said, "You have brain cancer."

**It felt like a tidal wave hit me. I didn't know how to
respond. I asked the doctor, "What are my odds?" He
said, "If you don't have the surgery, you have two weeks."**

Of course, I wanted to have the surgery. The doctors talked to my wife, whom I had just married two years earlier, and said I would be on disability the rest of my life. My brain surgery was set for April 26, 2005, just four days later.

I remember going to surgery praying to God that I would have the ability to talk and function when I came out. My brain surgery was eight hours. The neurosurgeon took out a cancerous grapefruit-sized, 8-centimeter mass. It was diagnosed as a grade 3, mixed oligoastrocytoma (a mixed glioma). I awoke from surgery very thirsty and confused. The stitches in my head made me look like Frankenstein.

I was discharged on May 2, 2005 and returned home.

Protocol and Pessimistic Prognosis

The doctors said, "We need to do the standard protocol." Twelve cycles of Temodar (a pill), and lots of other medications totaling twelve drugs at the same time. They all had many side effects, including the steroids that made me angry and hungry.

My teeth hurt when I ate, due to other medications. I gained a lot of weight and I couldn't sleep well. I was a physical and mental mess, often half awake. The side effects were often worse than what they were treating.

I also had radiation between June 6, 2005 and July 20, 2005. I developed "chemo brain." I felt slow and lethargic. It was hard to find the right words when speaking and I had short-term memory loss. I had a very hard time functioning and had to relearn how to organize everything in my life.

A couple of doctors were very negative and pessimistic about my prognosis. Statistically, the research showed that other people who had a similar cancer had a very poor prognosis. Deep down I knew the impact this could have on my life.

**I felt like a man standing on top of a tall cliff looking
over the edge at the age of 30, thinking this might be the
end of my life. I felt like I was walking on thin ice.**

After undergoing chemotherapy (Temodar) and radiation, I went back to work and slowly began to reassemble the broken pieces of my life.

Making Changes with Jeanne Wallace, Ph.D.

Along the way, I was fortunate to have found two brain tumor mentors, both of whom had glioblastomas. Someone who has "walked in your shoes" can be very helpful. One day, one of them said, "You need to talk to Jeanne Wallace." I learned that Jeanne Wallace, Ph.D., is one of the foremost experts in the nutritional cancer world.

I started to work with Jeanne in 2007. She said my outcome would be better if I changed my diet; she was very instrumental in helping me change it. I had been diagnosed as borderline diabetic, eating lots of fast food and other junk with lots of sugar. With her encouragement and recommendations, supported by evidence-based studies that she constantly researches, I drastically reduced my sugar intake, stopped drinking soda pop and learned to eat, primarily a green diet.

Jeanne had me get certain blood work every six months. From the results of the blood work, she continually made (and continues to make) a variety of treatment recommendations. She was always fact based in her recommendations. Jeanne also produced a substantial, factual, well-researched report about helpful supplements, dietary changes and how various studies confirmed how these things could help. Facts, not fluff, and compassion are a major part of her and her team's approach.

Now, I am only taking one pharmaceutical drug, but I continue to take 37 non-pharmaceutical pills, including 12 different vitamins, extracts, botanicals, and other supplements per day. I continue to have my blood drawn every six months and, as a result of the changes in my blood work, Jeanne and her team tweak my supplement protocol. We talk online or via phone consults. I also continue to have brain scans, about once per year.

I don't think I would be here today without Jeanne Wallace's well researched recommendations and protocol. Also, my faith has been instrumental. It helps me find purpose and meaning in life.

I grew up an evangelical Christian. Realizing I could die, I needed to set my affairs in order. My faith in God grew stronger as a result of this experience. I came to God with questions like, "Why me?"

That kind of question can bring about two outcomes. First, you may shake your fist at God in anger, or second, you may find purpose from the experience. There is a relationship between God and us. God is molding us throughout life. There is growth through suffering. Faith has helped me find purpose and meaning in this whole cancer journey.

Brain cancer involves your mind, body and spirit. Mentally, you must be engaged, you must keep the fight, you can't lose the fight, mentally or emotionally. Doctors only look at the physical issues, but what needs to be addressed are not the symptoms as much as the underlying cause. To survive and thrive with this you must keep your whole being strong and engaged. My faith has increased during my cancer fight and it has been my stronghold.

I have had a very supportive wife and parents through this journey. Now, I am working full time and look at myself as a "phoenix rising from the ashes," slowly rising up, one step at a time.

> Joshua quoted from the Bible, Psalm 139:14: "We are fearfully (awesomely) and wonderfully made." He went on to say, "How intricately our bodies are put together by the Maker."

Transformation and Pearls of Wisdom

It is important to live in the moment, enjoy what you have. I used to be negative and self-absorbed. Having cancer turns your whole world upside down. I was like John Wayne: I believed I could handle anything by myself. There is no place for pride when you have cancer. Cancer has made me more compassionate about other people's problems and issues. During the past two to three years, I have felt much better.

Mentors and caregivers can be very helpful, and they helped me greatly. I would not be here today without them. We all need support. Personally, I have mentored approximately 10 other people with cancer through Jonny Imerman's non-profit program, Imerman's Angels, which introduces people who are fighting cancer to others (angels) who have walked in their shoes and successfully fought the same kind of cancer.

Anyone recently diagnosed needs to find supportive and compassionate people to hold their hand through this; many resources are out there. Finding programs like Inheritance of Hope or First Descents (these are adventure retreats meant to empower and inspire) that help build you up for the fight ahead, and unite you with others, is critical.

Cancer is a big, grim topic; you are staring death in the face. It is about the Grim Reaper. When you are diagnosed, you want answers.

> **You become a new person when you are told you have cancer. It is a new normal, but you are not your cancer so don't let cancer become your identity.**

Allow yourself to cope, and find a good support network. Strangely, cancer has been a blessing, because it has allowed me to see the world in a whole new way and enjoy every moment I have left. I wouldn't trade it for anything.

> **Find things for yourself that can bring you peace. Find purpose, because many things don't make sense. It takes time. Find strength. You can feel like the ground is breaking up under your feet, but there is hope. Live in the moment.**

There are other things beyond the conventional and standard protocols that can be very helpful like Jeanne Wallace's program and people with similar protocols like hers. However, you must be careful about what you believe on the Internet. There are some snake oil salespeople out there. You must be discerning and become an advocate for yourself.

Joshua closed with this quote from the book *AntiCancer: A New Way of Life*, by Dr. David Servan-Screiber: "...lifestyle choices play on our genes like a pianist's fingers on a keyboard ... transforming the body's ability to resist cancer growth."

PART TWO

Exclusive Interviews with Five Renowned Cancer Specialists
and How They Are Saving Lives Now

About Part Two This section is comprised of interviews I conducted with five renowned doctors and healthcare practitioners who look at cancer somewhat differently from their conventional colleagues.

These individuals are viewed in their realm as true icons—veritable difference makers, trailblazers and thought leaders—all engaged in groundbreaking clinical work. They are researchers, educators, and hands-on practitioners with vast clinical experience. Some of these practitioners treat patients with a highly personalized, integrative therapeutic philosophy, while others apply alternative treatments and therapies.

They offer unvarnished opinions about the cancer industry, including candid views of novel treatments, therapies, and research. Their unique perspectives—coupled with the efficacy of their treatment modalities and exceptional outcomes compared to the strict "standard of care"—are deeply thought provoking.

Remember, "standard of care" predominantly refers to conventional treatments: surgery, chemotherapy and radiation therapy, as well as hormonal therapy, as the primary tools utilized in fighting cancer.

These five practitioners courageously think outside the box and expand the toolbox of conventional cancer treatments and therapies with innovative, efficacious, safe, evidence-based protocols. They have saved many lives in their practices, and continue to save the lives of many people who were considered terminal and beyond the scope of conventional treatment.

The interviews that follow are with five of the most renowned and respected experts in the integrative and alternative cancer world. It has been my privilege to be afforded the unique opportunity to inquire, directly, about their viewpoints and attitudes. Their opinions and thoughts are replete with unique insights, wisdom, practical advice, and deeply informed courses of action.

KEITH BLOCK, M.D.

ABOUT KEITH BLOCK, M.D. Keith I. Block, M.D., is an internationally recognized expert in integrative oncology. Referred to by many as the "father of integrative oncology," Dr. Block combines cutting-edge conventional treatments with individualized and scientifically based complementary and nutraceutical therapies. In 1980, he co-founded the Block Center for Integrative Cancer Treatment in Skokie, Illinois, the first such facility in North America, and serves as its medical and scientific director.

The field of integrative oncology was formally recognized by the launching of Integrative Cancer Therapies (ICT). In 2000, Dr. Block was invited by Sage Science Press to be the founding editor-in-chief of this peer-reviewed journal; the first medical journal devoted to exploring the research and science behind integrative oncology. In 2007, ICT was accepted by Thomson Scientific for inclusion in the Science Citation Index Expanded™.

Dr. Block is the scientific director of the Institute for Integrative Cancer Research and Education, where he has collaborated with colleagues at the University of Illinois at Chicago, the University of Texas MD Anderson Cancer Center in Houston and Bar Ilan University in Israel. Dr. Block is also on Dr. Andrew Weil's faculty at the Arizona Center for Integrative Medicine at the University of Arizona College of Medicine.

In 2005, he was appointed to the National Cancer Institute's Physician Data Query (PDQ) Cancer CAM editorial board, on which he continues to serve today.

Dr. Block has more than 120 publications in scientific journals and books relevant to nutritional and integrative oncology. He is also the author of Life Over Cancer, published by Bantam Books in 2009.

His model of individualized integrative oncology continues to set the standard for the practice of this comprehensive approach to cancer treatment in the U.S.

Interview

Q: What impelled you to become seriously involved in a comprehensive integrative cancer practice as opposed to a conventional "standard of care" practice?

A: I had three relatives who died of cancer when I was growing up. My uncle died when I was 8 years old, my grandfather when I was 12, and my grandmother had a breast cancer recurrence when I was 14. I remember going to the hospital to visit her with my parents.

This was a robust, charismatic woman who had been receiving chemotherapy, and had become debilitated, depleted and was clearly in despair. Her doctors were so focused on eradicating the disease, that no one addressed her nutrition to combat her depleted state; no one considered her debilitation and muscle wasting by encouraging any physical therapy or even basic rebuilding; and no one was paying any attention to her despair by providing support and helping her deal with understandable emotional needs.

Intuitively, this made absolutely no sense to me, and she eventually died from cancer cachexia (a wasting syndrome faced by many cancer patients). I'm sure that on some subconscious level, this experience was a driving force that led me into the cancer world. Certainly, it was instrumental in steering me toward introducing lifestyle interventions for patients and in developing the first integrative cancer treatment center before it was the "in" thing to do.

When I went to medical school I had no immediate intention to go into oncology. I was an athlete throughout my youth and early college years, and had what one might call unconventional ideas about the potential of the human organism, leaning towards an interest in disease prevention and health. As a kid, I was fascinated by people who took on extreme, impressive physical challenges. My boyhood heroes included people who accomplished extraordinary feats—like Chuck Yeager, who broke the sound barrier; Edmund Hillary and Tenzing Norgay, the two mountaineers who successfully climbed Mount Everest; and Ernest Shackleton and his crew, who survived the brutal winter elements while trapped in Antarctica—to name a few.

The appeal of these feats—that is, exceeding what had already been accomplished, reaching for what might be possible— would ultimately become fundamental in my approach to patient care and an underlying principle of our integrative practice.

My own health challenges in medical school made me keenly aware of the scarcity of treatment options available in the conventional medicine world. I knew there had to be something beyond the limitations I encountered in conventional medicine, and it was these experiences that sent me down the path of what would ultimately come to be universally known as "integrative" cancer treatment.

Early on during my medical training I remember carrying cancer cells from one lab to another, just a short 30 yards down the hall, to a graduate student in a second lab. He was quite impatient, yelling for me to move faster, because the cells would likely die during this short walk, preventing him from doing his lab work.

While racing back to get another batch of malignant cells, I found myself shaking my head, confused and troubled. How had these cancer cells that could not survive a simple quick walk, wreak such havoc in the human body, that they killed my uncle, grandfather and grandmother by the time I turned 16?

The contrast was instructive. Detached from their surroundings, separated from the body and their microenvironment, cancer cells are actually quite fragile and vulnerable. A light bulb went off in my mind as I realized that our bodies should have the ability to coddle or combat cancer, depending on the state or condition of our biochemical environment, which is the environment these cells reside in.

Cancer patient survival is as much about integrative and nutritional interventions, even when pertaining to advanced disease, as it is about the disease itself. Innovative approaches and individualizing treatments to each patient's condition, biology, biochemical and molecular profile are critical to care, and this is a significant driving force in both our diagnostic and treatment methodologies.

When implementing conventional therapies that have considerable toxicity, it is essential to have a patient in the best shape possible to tolerate treatment better, and to respond more favorably.

I am in the business of saving lives!

Those of us who have clinical careers that are directed toward helping those who are facing a fragile future would certainly rather have our patients be in better condition when we begin treatment. There's not a single surgeon, or at least there shouldn't be, who wouldn't rather have their patient more physically, nutritionally, emotionally and biologically fit, before carting them off to the operating room. Why should this be any different for a cancer specialist? This is simple common sense.

Patients with better performance status, a medical term for assessing a patient's general condition, do better in every aspect. They tolerate treatments better, respond better, have better life quality and better outcomes and survival.

Q: I've heard you say we have made some recent gains, but overall, and for many years, we have been losing the "war on cancer." Why do you believe this is the case?

A: Other than Hodgkin's disease, some childhood cancers and some recent changes among a few less common cancers, the actual change in cancer mortality over the past 65 years has been less than five percent.

Contrast this 5 percent with other major diseases such as cardiovascular disease and stroke. There's been an approximate 64 percent decrease in deaths from cardiovascular disease and a 74 percent decrease in the number of deaths from strokes over this same period of time.

Why this significant discrepancy in decreased mortality?

For the answer, we need to look no further than our current conventional model of cancer treatment. We talk in our culture as if screening is prevention.

Screenings—such as colonoscopies, mammograms, prostate exams, routine dermatological evaluation and other screening methodologies—are not true prevention.

Screening is catching it after it's caught you. True prevention is stopping cancer before it catches you!

While screening is important, and catching cancer early increases the odds of a favorable outcome, one shouldn't confuse screening with true prevention. And while we say things like "lose weight," "get fit with regular exercise," and "stop smoking," it is not core to our mainstream approach to medical care, and when it comes to cancer, these most basic lifestyle strategies are not remotely as prominent as they should be.

These recommendations are made as generic recommendations. In my opinion, the optimal cancer prevention model includes detailed assessments and evaluations that screen for biochemical disruptions and correct terrain imbalances.

Q: Philosophically, are you saying the strict "standard of care" approach versus a "comprehensive and personalized integrative approach" is quite different?

A: Yes, I am.

Mainstream cancer treatment grows out of a cultural, and global fixation on seeking out silver bullet treatment strategies. This search, while fruitful in small ways, has missed the bigger gains we might have made had we kept the individual as an important central aspect of the ensuing battle.

Instead, it's been displaced by the search for a powerful "Johnny-one-note," single drug solution. Matching a single drug to a single target has rarely worked at establishing a cure. This search and way of thinking are not limited to conventional care, but can be found among those practicing in the alternative and Complementary and Alternative Medicine (CAM) camps as well.

I believe much of the interest in discovering a single curative treatment grew out of our earlier historical experience with antibiotics. While single-use antibiotic treatments appeared to be successful early on, over time we have witnessed enormous antibiotic resistance, which has led to far more aggressive, antibiotic-resistant bacterial strains.

In a similar way, resistance has become an even greater problem for cancers and cancer drugs than it has with antibiotics. Yet, when we look at the history of cancer, we only rarely find a single drug or a single target intervention that does much more than temporarily slow growth. Even when we do, it is mostly limited to a few months.

In spite of a large marketing effort touting "personalized care," most treatment is about matching one drug to a molecular biomarker, and not comprehensively individualizing treatment based on objective criteria, including nutrition, physical care, bio-behavioral, metabolic and molecular profiling. Such profiling provides our center with a means for modifying care to comprehensively formulating a treatment plan that is genuinely individualized at every aspect of treatment and care.

The fact is, a single molecular site does not represent the full vulnerability of a cancer, the Achilles heel of the cancer. Rather, cancer growth is driven by a group of intersecting critical growth tracts. Thus, for improving one's odds for attaining genuine success with treatment, we take a different approach. In order to broadly analyze multiple targets and growth tracts of a patient's cancer, we use several different technologies and with the results, we map out a group of multi-targeted strategies in order to more comprehensively and individually address the complexity associated with cancer growth.

Certainly, there have been considerable gains in recent years with experimental treatment approaches including molecular, angiogenic and immune-based therapies. However, though some lip service is given to these, most mainstream treatment approaches exist without a foundation of health. Thus, they lack the fundamentals essential for reversing, slowing or containing tumor growth, improving tolerance, diminishing toxicity and enhancing treatment sensitivity.

In my experience, implementing a tailored regimen in order to build a foundation of optimal health is essential to acquiring a successful outcome.

Also, it is important to note that patients rarely die from cancer, but rather from disease or treatment-related complications. With an aggressive lifestyle regimen focused on personalized nutritional-oncology care, a physical rebuilding and maintenance program designed to address the patient's clinical status, and a bio-behavioral regimen tailored to the patient's needs, it is possible to prevent the onset or counter the impact of these complications. These problems can include pneumonia, blood clots, emboli, wasting syndromes and sepsis, among others.

As we compare integrative cancer treatment to conventional options, definitions become more important in order to understand what is being advised and what is needed.

From my viewpoint, the definition of alternative therapy is treatment offered in lieu of mainstream therapy, and may lack rigorous evidence. I think most CAM is really a haphazard set of single intervention "add-ons." For example, green tea with prostate cancer treatment, or yoga for breast cancer are "add-ons." They are not systematic approaches to care any more than most mainstream care is systematic.

When it comes to defining integrative treatment, most centers have framed it around the use of mostly generic multiple treatment modalities. Along with CAM, this too often provides complementary, generic, single intervention therapies, doled out without the precision basis of systematized care. This shortchanges the patient from a myriad of perspectives.

**Core to my philosophy of care (as is detailed in
my book, Life Over Cancer), the treatment of
cancer must be a '...systematic, comprehensive,
multi- intervention, whole systems model with
treatment strategies individualized to the patient,
based upon objective assessments, provided
with a life-affirming and open communication
between patients and practitioners.'**

This is how I define true integrative cancer treatment, a model I hope and
believe will one day be far more broadly embraced and implemented.

**Q: Some cancer centers have opened integrative departments with a
naturopathic doctor or perhaps one integrative medical doctor, but I
wonder if these initiatives truly incorporate the comprehensive complementary, personalized treatments and therapies you recommend? Do
you have an opinion about this?**

A: This is a tricky question, because I don't want to undermine what are
positive steps that some cancer centers have begun taking. Some of these
centers make complementary therapies available, but they're not systematically
integrated into a comprehensive program. Nor are they tailored to meet each
patient's specific needs.

In other words, just because there may be a massage table down the hall from
a chemotherapy unit, it does not mean the facility provides a true comprehensive, integrative oncology program.

Q: How does a patient's lifestyle and diet impact cancer?

A: The data and studies looking at the relationship between nutrition
and cancer are voluminous. However, there is a major disconnect between
what is evidence based and supported by the literature, and what the average

mainstream clinician is comfortable with when it comes to advising patients who are battling for their lives.

For many years now, the American Cancer Society and other institutions have talked about the wise preventive strategy of cutting back on cancer-promoting lifestyle choices. However, once a patient gets diagnosed with cancer, that message disappears and is replaced by the well intentioned, though seriously misguided, "eat whatever you want."

This advice grows out of a mindset that encourages patients to eat foods which are calorically dense but nutrient poor, high in saturated fats and simple and refined carbohydrates, such as milk shakes, red meat, ice cream, canned and processed foods.

This is particularly problematic when it comes to combating weight loss, a cancer-driven inflammatory condition that diminishes appetite, wastes muscle, and promotes further malignant growth.

Unfortunately, these calorically dense regimens can actually feed the patient's cancer, promoting malnutrition, and contributing to the patient's inability to tolerate treatment. In addition, if the malnutrition is not addressed, it can lead to a macronutrient deficit leading to a condition called "cachexia," defined as a wasting syndrome that results in compromised immunity, weakness, and a loss of weight, body fat, and muscle.

As a starting point, our diets, our sedentary life, high levels of unrelieved stress, toxic relationships and sleep disruption, all lay the groundwork for not only getting cancer, but for driving cancer forward.

For example, there is good research for solid tumor cancers, showing that exercise and fitness, speed walking 45 to 60 minutes per day, can reduce cancer mortality by 50 percent!

In years gone by, in my grandmother's era certainly, and even throughout my own training, doctors told cancer patients to "go home and rest." I have resisted this thinking for nearly 40 years. One needs a balance between activity and rest. You need to sleep well to have the vitality to be active during the day. And generally speaking, the more active you are during the day, the better you will sleep at night.

Activity and rest cycles are essential for establishing a healthy and optimal circadian rhythm. Additionally, since fatigue is so heavily associated with cancer and its treatments, strategies for improving circadian health are of utmost priority.

Regarding weight gain, for example, studies show that just five kilograms (11 pounds) of extra weight can increase mortality in breast cancer by 14 percent! It should be noted, with some cancers, that it is not uncommon for people undergoing chemotherapy to gain weight. This weight gain is clearly associated with higher recurrence risk and poorer outcomes. In addition, patients who are obese, regardless of the type of cancer, generally have a higher mortality than patients who have normal body weight.

Regarding the impact of diet, it is clear that the typical Western diet can drive the onset of malignancy. For example, according to several studies, red meat can increase the risk of colorectal cancer by 35 to 85 percent, and the risk of pancreatic cancer by 25 to 75 percent.

Also, high milk and calcium consumption are associated with a 15 to 200 percent increase in prostate cancer. And one randomized controlled trial showed that when breast cancer patients reduced their fat intake to 20 percent or lower, they reduced their risk of recurrence by an average of 24 percent! This is on par with Tamoxifen, which has shown a 25 percent reduction in recurrence rates after taking it for five years.

Today, we tell patients with hormone-sensitive cancers to take hormonal blockers for 10 plus years, and that they will get a 50 percent reduction of recurrence, but no one has done a comparable study with dietary intake to see about the reduction of recurrence if you are eating healthfully for 10 years.

There is also impressive data showing that if you shift to a whole grain, legume based, vegetable and fruit diet, you cut back cancer risks dramatically, yet there is probably less than a three percent chance that your cancer specialist will bring up a discussion about diet with you!

This is remarkable, given the supporting evidence for making dietary changes. Another example: 25 grams of flax per day will cut your Ki67, a proliferation marker for cancer, by 34 percent. There is also evidence to suggest that 25 grams of flaxseed per day can induce apoptosis (the normal, genetically-regulated process of cell death) by 30 percent. Yet, we don't talk about nutrition specificity as a medical culture.

We can counter the risk of cancers by controlling and countering exposure to [cancer cell] growth stimulants. We know that body weight, dietary fats and refined flours and sugars will drive up insulin growth factors, increase the surge of insulin and insulin resistance, driving cancers forward. Additionally, various stressors can lead to insulin resistance, thus raising the output of insulin with potential [cancer cell] growth inducing consequences.

Even basic things like a drop in albumin and protein levels are associated with the inability of cancer patients to fight off infections. If you look at the low albumin levels of cancer patients in any hospital, you would find a large percentage suffer from marked albuminemia. Most conventional medicine doctors would say, "Well, many of these patients are late stage; we can't feed them."

I don't buy it! We have taken many patients who, when they first came to us, had moderate to marked cachexia and laboratory-confirmed inflammatory problems, in large part because they were fed high calorie "corporate shakes," which are loaded with both refined sugars and the wrong fats. This drives a pro-inflammatory condition even further, leading to muscle wasting and appetite suppression. If you change those fats to healthier fats and add complex carbohydrates, you change the inflammatory cascade and suddenly these patients are able to start eating again. You rebuild their proteins, their albumin level and muscle mass and they'll become active again. It does not happen all at once or for all patients, but I can tell you from firsthand experience, a large percentage of these patients will respond and turn around.

I think our ignorance and lack of attention to nutrition and integrative care in general hastens not only the disease process, but also the dying process.

I would argue nutritional therapy should be standard of care, but supplementation must be designed from careful clinical evaluation and from comprehensive terrain and metabolic laboratory panels, enabling individualized recommendations for each patient.

Q: Let's talk about chemotherapy for a few minutes. Before you engage in chemotherapy treatments do you recommend patients obtain chemosensitivity testing of tissue samples?

A: One of the most critical decisions that cancer doctors help patients make is determining which chemotherapy regimen is likely to work best. There are often many options with no clear-cut reason to choose one over another. Occasionally, existing research data may help a doctor lean toward one regimen, but this rarely addresses the individual's unique biology and tumor characteristics.

Chemotherapy works brilliantly for a few patients, pretty well for some and poorly or not at all for others. This holds true even for people with the same stage of the same cancer.

Every cancer is unique; breast cancer is not a single disease, nor is colon or pancreatic cancer or any other kind of cancer. The art of cancer treatment is to determine which set of chemotherapies or molecular target drugs has the most likely chance of countering malignant growth.

Genomic and proteomic testing provide information on growth pathways and molecular characteristics of a patient's disease. Chemotherapy-sensitivity assays (testing) help determine which drugs the patient's own cancer tissue is most sensitive to. By exploring and testing drugs with a patient's tissue in the lab, it becomes easier to determine what the best match of a particular chemotherapy protocol or targeted drug would be before trying it out on the patient. This can lead to less exposure to ineffective drugs and better odds for selecting the right drugs, with better overall response, remission and survival.

Yes, when you have the ability to test tissue, it definitely should be done.

> **Dr. Robert Nagourney's groundbreaking work has provided an invaluable tool in the task of selecting optimal chemotherapy regimens for patients. His work offers doctors a method to better select drugs that are more likely to work on an individual patient's cancer, while avoiding unnecessary protocols that may not work as well, and worse, may cause adverse side effects.**

Dr. Nagourney's recognition of the importance of the microenvironment is a point of distinction of his testing methodology. His assay is the only method I'm aware of where the potential effectiveness of a drug is evaluated against the cancer cell in the context of its microenvironment—the tumor stroma or matrix, blood vessels, and inflammatory cells—where the cancer cells reside. When a tumor sample arrives at the Rational Therapeutics laboratory, it is broken up into "micro-spheroids," fragments that preserve the tumor along with its surroundings. Dr. Nagourney and his staff then test drugs in a situation closer to real-life biology than other chemosensitivity tests. Their team will test numerous chemotherapeutic drugs as well as drug combinations against the patient's actual tissue sample.

As opposed to what is being called personalized medicine, a more comprehensive use of these tests, along with individualizing each component of an integrative program to each patient, provides a true tailored and personalized approach to clinical care.

Q: I understand one of your chemotherapeutic infusion and distribution techniques is unique in the United States. I am referring to chronomodulated chemotherapeutic treatments. How does this methodology work?

A: Back in the early nineties, I was looking for methods to help my patients better tolerate some of the more invasive cancer treatments. When I came across some of the research of Bill Hrushevsky, M.D., clearly the pioneer in the field of chronomodulated chemotherapy, it was a light bulb moment for me. Dr. Hrushevsky suggests his work demonstrates a substantial reduction in adverse effects, in some cases up to an 85 percent reduction. It turns out that most every drug has an optimal time of day or night when it is most effective and least toxic. By administering drugs during this time, there is substantial evidence demonstrating greater treatment response and improved outcomes.

Other evidence demonstrates you can re-challenge a patient with the same exact drug protocol that they had not responded to or stopped responding to previously, and by chronomodulating the administration of the drug you can attain an improved response rate among 40-50 percent of the patients.

It is not simply the timing, but also the style of the infusion based on what is referred to as a sinusoidal wave. The pump initially infuses the drug in very small increments. Then slowly and methodically, the amount of drug is administered at an increasing rate until a peak concentration is reached. Then, the infusion is slowly reduced, until the remaining drug has been fully administered. Providing the drug in this manner requires special programmable infusion pumps.

It turns out that we have nine specific clock-related genes that control a great deal of our biological functioning, including sleeping, eating patterns, heart rate, body temperature, hormonal production and others. Cancer cells and the drugs used to treat them have their own time control.

Optimally, cancer drugs should be administered at the precise time when specific cancer cells are dividing and are more vulnerable to cell death. Fortunately, this is the same time when healthy cells have the least sensitivity to toxicity from chemotherapy. Thus, getting the timing and the style of administration of a patient's cancer drugs right is critical for optimizing the best response and outcome with the least adverse effects.

> **The fact is, the timing of drug administration, called chronotherapy, can markedly reduce chemotherapy treatment toxicity as well as show an impressive improvement in five-year survivals among those battling advanced cancer.**

In the last 25 years, it has been a very rare occasion that a new drug for advanced cancer patients has shown more than a two to four month improvement in median survival. By timing the administration of chemotherapy, one can also improve treatment tolerance, have a profound impact on a patient's response to treatment, and improve outcome and clinical results while boosting overall survival.

With such significant benefits, one might ask why chronotherapy isn't routine among cancer centers. Unfortunately, in spite of the benefits, there is no conventional reimbursement from either commercial insurance or Medicare for the expense of setting up a center with this innovative technology, or for the expense incurred for the considerable training required.

Mainstream centers schedule patients for chemotherapy around the doctor's schedule. However, providing chemotherapy in a center that provides chronotherapy would require the doctors to schedule themselves around the patient and their treatment schedule.

Research has demonstrated that approximately 25 to 35 percent of patients discontinue chemotherapy treatment prematurely due to debilitating psychological and physical consequences of treatment. We believe the interventions of chronomodulated chemotherapeutic administration, combined with integrative care and intravenous nutrition, provide significant value to patients. We also provide detoxifying compounds to mitigate toxic metabolites from the chemotherapeutic drugs, because toxic metabolites contribute to drug resistance, toxicity and mutations. These toxic metabolites make cancer cells more aggressive, and the treatment less effective.

While this treatment is common in Europe and available in the Mideast and Asia, today, our center is the only one in the U.S. administering chemotherapeutic drugs in a chronomodulated fashion. It is costly to set up a treatment unit to administer chronomodulated chemotherapy and, as covered earlier, there is no reimbursement or additional compensation from insurance or Medicare for the expense in setting up a treatment unit like ours. This is in spite of the considerable savings from less toxicity, better treatment tolerance and improved outcomes.

The medical oncology community is driven primarily by introducing new drugs, but not by the timing, style and method that they are infused. Nor are they interested in the many low cost agents that can improve tolerance and outcome. Thus, it is unfortunate that with our knowledge that chemotherapies have an optimal timing when they are the least toxic and the most treatment sensitive, there isn't much drive and interest to attend to how these drugs are administered.

Q: The issue of using antioxidants during chemotherapy has been debated for a long time. Your thoughts?

A: Without a doubt, without any doubt, considerable studies demonstrate that a broad range of natural agents, antioxidants, and vitamins can be helpful to mitigate chemotherapeutic toxicity and enhance response and outcome.

Many of these studies are smaller, mostly because there are only limited funds for research of this kind. The available funds for research are generally limited due to low interest in agents and compounds that are difficult to, or simply cannot be, patented.

For example, randomized controlled trials on ginger used for delaying nausea and vomiting are fairly well accepted. Anti-inflammatory trials demonstrating the benefits of American and Korean ginseng are well known and commonplace. Also, there are trials supporting the efficacy of L-carnitine, in preventing treatment-related cardiotoxicity. There is evidence of the use of vitamin E and CoQ10 protecting the heart from cardiomyopathy caused by anthracyclines. We also know vitamin E has been used with taxanes and platinum to reduce neuropathy.

Additionally, there are trials supporting the benefits of limited periods of use for glutamine and other agents in dealing with the effects of mucositis and mouth sores caused by 5-FU. To counter radiation burns, there are trials clearly supporting the use of calendula.

Q: I've heard you speak often about the importance of the "biochemical terrain." How does our terrain influence our risk of getting cancer?

A: I have spent the past 30 years investigating the clinical relevance and influence that the extracellular and intracellular environments have on cancer cells. A patient's biochemical terrain can either be cancer promoting or cancer inhibiting.

If a more comprehensive lab assessment is performed, one that includes oxidative, inflammatory, immune, nutritional, and other relevant biomarkers, the results can provide a direction for clinical intervention. A patient's terrain can be favorably modified through the use of nutritional and off-label medications. Our testing provides an "objective fingerprint" allowing for individualized intervention.

For example, immune suppression due to treatment such as chemotherapy, nutritional deficiencies, emotional despair or the disease itself, can have profound negative effects on a patient's overall condition as well as their ability to tolerate and respond to treatment.

Similarly, if your inflammatory markers are elevated and cancer cells secrete inflammatory chemistry, you become pro-inflammatory from the disease. Additionally, you can become pro-inflammatory from the typical Western diet, sleep disruption, and stress. Most people sitting in hospitals do not get measured for C-reactive protein, fibrinogen sedimentation rates, interleukin-2

and other markers associated with inflammation. Getting a detailed understanding of the patient's status, prior to starting treatment, can have a significant impact on outcome. We need to set a solid foundation first.

Toxicity and side effects are directly correlated. If you have a high oxidative stressed environment from diet, stress and conventional therapies, this
oxidative stress propels the environment. It affects tumor growth, brings
about side effects, and impacts quality of life. In addition, drug resistance is
associated with this bio-chemical soup. This is the adverse side, as the soup
promotes oncogenes [genes with potential to cause cancer] and interrupts
tumor suppressor gene expression.

We "map" patients, and then do aggressive assessments in a comprehensive
way to get a "fingerprint" of their metabolic and molecular terrain, also known
as intracellular and intercellular terrain. We get blood and tissue. We intervene
first with natural agents if possible, because they are safer, less costly, and less
toxic, but we will also use approved drugs that have been demonstrated to
affect these particular targets.

There is a plethora of research showing that it is quite possible to create an
inhospitable microenvironment where cancer cells lose ground, where toxicity
is mitigated and the treatments work quite well. Laying a better foundation
helps patients do dramatically better in every facet. It is a fantasy to think
that a single strategy will be curative for a complex disease. Cancer requires a
multi-targeted model and a multi-dimensional approach. Integrative medicine
must include whole-patient thinking.

**We look for actionable targets, not just one or two
targets associated with the disease, which drugs do. We
look to target, comprehensively, all the potential
Achilles heels of the disease.**

In 2009, there was a *Journal of Clinical Oncology* study that showed highly
elevated inflammatory markers in a large sample of breast cancer patients. The
patients who had the highest Serum Amyloid A (SAA) protein levels and high

C-reactive proteins (CRP) levels had a three to four times the rates of mortality and cancer recurrence. This is not at all surprising. Also, cancer patients with diabetes have about half the survival levels and a much higher rate of recurrence versus other cancer patients, due to the fact that cancer cells gobble up glucose at a remarkably higher rate than do normal cells.

Q: Is there anything patients can do once they've completed chemotherapy to help prevent a recurrence?

A: This is perhaps the most overlooked aspect of conventional oncology. Once a patient is deemed in remission, they are typically disconnected from care, as well as any attending support, and told to come back in three to six months where diagnostic scans or blood tests will determine if the cancer has returned. I suggest a far more proactive, empowered approach. For the past few decades I have developed a program for maintaining remission. Every patient that goes into remission deserves a remission maintenance plan that offers cancer survivors a personalized program to regain control of their health, restore vitality and protect against the cancer returning.

Once a patient has completed their treatment, we conduct an updated detailed integrative assessment, and then personally tailor a comprehensive remission maintenance program that includes a full detox plan in order to restore and rehabilitate from the prior treatment regimen. Following this, we update therapeutic nutrition, prescriptive exercise, bio-behavioral strategies, selective supplementation and anti-tumor therapies with the goal of sustaining long-term remission.

It is quite understandable that after a patient hears "You're in remission," their inclination is to psychologically retreat to a cancer-free zone and never think about cancer again. Not a good idea!

And here's why: Cancer is invisible, as much a microscopic and molecular disease as it is a visible one. Thus a patient in remission may still harbor malignant cells (ones that were resistant to chemotherapy or radiation, and therefore survived the "attack phase," or treatment phase). Unfortunately, these cells have the ability to return and show up with a vengeance, when a person least suspects it.

At the Block Center, particularly in the first year or two of remission, we provide "aggressive monitoring," which includes lab tests and imaging to detect early signs of a disrupted biochemistry, or a recurrence of disease. In the first years after remission, therefore, we recommend:

- Clinical visits with your oncologist, at least every three to four months in the first and second year and every six months for the next several years

- Scans and blood tests of tumor markers every three to four months

- Complete blood count and chemistry test every three months

- Updated integrative assessments including evaluating bio-behavioral, physical and nutrition status, including strength, flexibility, aerobic competence, weight changes, body composition, and albumin levels, every three months

- Internal comprehensive terrain monitoring, every three to six months for the terrain factors that are most potentially problematic

While doing this monitoring, there is no reason to simply wait anxiously for the proverbial other shoe to drop. We also immediately implement the remission maintenance program I referenced above. We know that people whose biochemical environments are disrupted have higher recurrence rates and greater mortality. Conversely, it's possible to keep the biochemical environment in harmony.

And the implementation of individualized, specific lifestyle interventions and dietary strategies can harness immune and biological defenses to help restore both physical and psychological vitality, as well as improve the odds of staying cancer-free.

Where recurrence risks are high, we will also carefully select immune and off-label treatment regimens appropriate to the disease and a patient's needs.

Q: How about stem cells? Any thoughts on how to kill cancer stem cells?

A: Everyone knows that there are things we do to treat cancer, but about two to five percent of every tumor is made up of cancer stem cells that work and function from different growth tracks.

We have been working hard to design different natural therapies and regimens to go after these stem cells. There are a number of drugs that are used—metformin is one example—that are off-label but work to strangulate sugar and insulin supply to cancer cells, and also block cancer stem cells.

In addition to off-label medications to fight cancer cells, my research team and I are presently working on additional strategies to fight stem cells. Unfortunately, I can't get into specifics at this time, due to the fact that it's in the preliminary testing phase.

Q: Do you have any golden nuggets or pearls of wisdom you would like to impart to the readers of this book who are facing a dire cancer prognosis?

A: One of the most common sources of distress after a diagnosis of cancer is being told that you have X number of months or years to live.

We have seen many patients over the years who were given a dire prognosis, who are doing extremely well many years later. Unfortunately, there is a premature fatalism that pervades much of cancer care.

This is often presented in the form of a risk-based percentage, such as "a 30 percent chance of surviving one year." For anyone on the receiving end of such a dire prediction, such statements can seem tantamount to a death sentence, often resulting in profound grief and depression. In fact, some patients simply stop fighting and caring for themselves. Instead of finding ways to live, they focus on preparing to die.

I urge my patients to resist these fatalistic communications. They can be prophetic and have physiologic impact. A terminal mindset can have terminal consequences; terrifying words from a medical authority the patient has come to respect can lead to a patient unintentionally fulfilling the prophecy.

For example, if told, "you have only six months to live," a patient may inadvertently develop the psychophysiology needed to fulfill the prediction. This can actually hasten the dying process and increase the odds of a terminal outcome! I suggest patients prepare for the worst and live for the best.

I'm aware that a patient is sometimes advised by a physician to avoid "false hope." But this misses the point altogether. First of all, hope can never be false. Hope is not a promise; rather it is a prayer! It is a prayer that can be followed with genuine action and integrative treatment in order to improve one's odds and potentially—hopefully—one's outcome!

In truth, I worry far more about patients receiving false hopelessness than false hope. False hope would run the risk of a communication of exaggerated expectations. But false hopelessness runs the risk of leaving a patient with excessive despair. It is despair and hopelessness that can hasten disease progression and drive death!

JEANNE WALLACE, PH.D., C.N.C.

ABOUT JEANNE WALLACE, PH.D., CNC Jeanne M. Wallace, Ph.D., CNC is widely regarded as a prominent international expert in nutritional oncology. She is the founder and director of Nutritional Solutions, which provides consulting to cancer patients throughout the U.S. and abroad, about evidence-based dietary, nutritional and botanical support to complement conventional cancer care.

Dr. Wallace completed her undergraduate studies magna cum laude at Boston University, earned her nutrition consulting degree at Bauman College in Santa Cruz, California, and completed her Ph.D. in nutrition through American State University. She is a member of the American Nutrition Association, has authored numerous articles, and lectured widely at cancer conferences and seminars for medical professionals.

Nutritional Solutions provides cutting-edge translational research in nutrition oncology and innovative cancer nutrition guidance to people with cancer and their families, as well as to healthcare practitioners such as oncologists, naturopaths, and other healthcare providers. She pioneered the oncometabolic approach to cancer nutrition in 1996, which is a cornerstone of her methodology.

Her trusted and uniquely qualified clinician, Michelle Gerencser, M.S., joined her later. Together, they have more than 35 years of clinical experience and continue to evolve their approach in response to emerging research.

Nutritional Solutions has served thousands of clients all over the world, consulting by phone and Skype. Easily digestible and comprehensive written materials, drawing on almost 9,000 published peer reviewed studies from biomedical journals, along with the one-on-one consulting relationship, allows each client to increase his or her cancer nutrition knowledge base, and a deep personal understanding of cancer nutrition as a manner of living. The deeply focused efforts of Dr. Wallace and her colleague, Michelle Gerencser, are grounded in the evolving understanding of the interrelationship between nutritional and metabolic factors, and the hallmark characteristics of cancer cells.

Dr. Wallace states, "Cancer cells do not exist in isolation; they are influenced by the environment within the body. Our goal is to teach our clients dietary and lifestyle strategies to modulate this environment, so that it is a less favorable host for tumor growth and progression. This approach is particularly well suited as a complement to conventional medical treatments for cancer, and allows our clients to optimize their care by integrating the best of both worlds."

Interview

Q: What motivated you to devote your career to nutritional, dietary and botanical research, including personal consultation and education for cancer patients?

A: My passion for this field was born of a significant family history of cancer, including colorectal, bladder, lung, pancreatic and gynecologic cancers, as well as malignant melanoma. I've lost dear friends and family members, been the caregiver for a friend with a brain tumor (now a survivor since 1997), and nurtured many loved ones on the path to long-term survivorship.

My mom is my hero, a Super-Duper-Double-Survivor, having beaten two different types of cancer (two unrelated primaries). Her first cancer diagnosis came during my freshman year in college and made a momentous impression on me. I'm fond of saying, "I didn't sign up for this; I was drafted."

These experiences have given my work in the field personal meaning and a sense of urgency. And this is true for all the members of our team. We've been personally impacted and we're on a mission to make a difference.

Q: Cancer is such a scary proposition. For many, it's a paralyzing and daunting foe. When and what inspired you with the belief that you could make a serious difference in people's lives?

A: I knew intimately the healing power of nutrition from my own experience restoring wellness after a health crisis in my mid-20s, an autoimmune condition for which the medical field had no cure, just symptom-suppressing 'band-aids.' I turned to nutrition and herbal medicine to successfully nourish myself back to health and experienced firsthand the potent healing power of whole foods fresh from the garden.

This prompted me to pursue a career in holistic nutrition (and to devote much of my free time to puttering in the garden). Early in my career, I gained a following in my community as someone who had an encyclopedic knowledge of how nutrition impacts health. People sought me out for help with their gout, cholesterol, allergies, colds, and a variety of other complaints. These early experiences showed me again and again how effective nutritional support could be in supporting the body's ability to rebuild health.

Cancer does seem scary and daunting when it's that monster-under-your-bed you hope you never have to confront. But when you or a loved one brings the diagnosis home, you're moved to act, to gather information, to understand your options—and all this brings empowerment to you.

In 1997, a dear friend was diagnosed with an aggressive brain tumor (a Glioblastoma Multiforme, grade IV). At the time, I was working with breast and ovarian cancers. Brain cancer did seem too scary. I looked for a referral, someone experienced in nutrition and brain tumors. There was no one, and I realized I'd been "drafted" yet again.

I tackled the literature and developed the first nutrition support plan for brain tumor clients. Despite a recurrence six months after her original diagnosis, she is alive and well today and has also survived breast cancer—so she's another Super-Duper-Double-Survivor in my life.

Q: Can you describe the fundamental tenets that form the foundation of your practice and consultative perspectives?

A: For us, it's not enough to provide expert knowledge in nutritional oncology. We're dedicated to serving our clients with compassion, empathy, respect, and kindness.

We understand the challenges of a cancer diagnosis, treatment, and recovery. Our consulting team listens with an understanding and appreciation of a client's situation. We respect each client's dignity, autonomy, and needs. Throughout life, each of us has cultivated an innate wisdom about our body. Our desire is to teach about wellness strategies that honor this wisdom and empower the client to make his/her own health choices. As our clients embark on their healing journeys, we strive to fill them with resilience, inspire them with hope, and empower them with confidence.

> **"No matter how scientifically advanced the practice of medicine becomes, true healing will always need to be combined with compassion."** ~Sogyal Rinpoche

Q: I have heard you mention an interesting term you've coined: "Oncometabolic Milieu." What does this mean? How is it relevant to cancer patients?

A: First, consider the words of these two great thinkers:

> **"It's more important to know what sort of person has a disease than to know what sort of disease a person has."** ~Hippocrates

"The art of healing comes from nature, not from the physician. Therefore, the physician must start from nature, with an open mind." ~Paracelsus

Let me answer with an analogy from biodynamic gardening, a hobby of mine. Let's say a colony of hungry aphids attacks a tree in your orchard of rare and heirloom fruits, say your prize Elephant Heart plum tree. One approach would be to spray pesticides—or organic versions thereof—to kill the aphids. But let's explore the situation deeper to see what answers nature can provide.

We know that a healthy garden ecosystem depends on several interdependent factors: sunlight, water, and healthy soil, to name a few. Within the soil live dense populations of beneficial fungi, which colonize the surface area of plant roots. These fungi convert minerals in the soil into bio-absorbable forms and help transport these nutrients into the plant's roots. To nourish the fungi, soil needs to have adequate carbohydrates (e.g., organic matter). If a plant is growing in soil deficient in organic matter, the soil will be devoid of beneficial fungi, and the plant will suffer from nutrient deficiencies no matter how much N-P-K fertilizer is applied.

A sickly tree appears particularly appetizing to aphids, which arrive in droves. Here's the amazing thing: the aphids, busily munching away, cause the plant's carbohydrate-rich sap to drip onto the soil below. This sap will seep into the soil, attract and feed the soil fungi, ultimately nourishing the plant back to health and halting further aphid activity. The organic-minded gardener can simply support the soil fungi by improving the soil. The aphid problem resolves itself, and the wise gardener is rewarded with award-winning plums.

It's not a quick fix as a blast of pesticides might be, but it's certainly an eloquent solution, one that corrects the underlying imbalances and works with rather than against nature.

Like aphids in the garden, cancer cells don't exist in isolation; their behavior is influenced by the environment within the body.

The Oncometabolic Milieu is the swirling sea of hormones, cytokines, eicosanoids, nutrients, growth factors, and signaling molecules that continually bathes and communicates with our cells. Indeed, this milieu modulates the oncogenic potential of cells and governs the ebb and flow of malignant behavior.

The time has come to relinquish our myopic view of "the tumor" and its innate characteristics in favor of a wider view that encompasses the full dynamic ecology of the human body. So think of the Oncometabolic Milieu as the soil, sun, water, and entire ecosystem exerting their influence on cancer cells.

Q: Can you describe how food may help or harm cancer patients in their attempt to fight cancer? Or, perhaps I should ask how food may strengthen or weaken a cancer patient's innate anti-cancer defenses?

A: Well foremost, one's diet significantly impacts the Oncometabolic Milieu. A diet that fosters systemic inflammation, insulin resistance, excess blood viscosity, nutrient imbalances and immune suppression will have a permissive effect with malignant cells. So, contrarily, our primary goal is to lessen these factors and create an internal environment that is not conducive to cancer growth and progression.

Most exciting is the discovery that our diet has direct effects on cancer genes. We've learned that genes are more plastic than originally thought. Gene expression is not written in stone; we're not stuck with the genetic-luck-of-the-draw with which we're born.

While we can't change the actual gene, we do have significant influence over which genes are expressed and which are kept dormant. This is accomplished via epigenetic 'marks,' regulatory machinery positioned on the surface of genes that controls which genes get turned on or off.

Consider this: Any single cell in your body carries the full set of genetic blueprints to build every organ in your body. So a single lung cell, for example, contains the genetic "recipes" for making a liver, eyeball, toenail, heart and brain. But only the blueprints needed to build a healthy lung and orchestrate its function are being expressed (hopefully). It is the epigenome that governs this.

Research in nutritional epigenetics is revealing how—at the molecular and genetic level—various anti-cancer foods repress the expression of oncogenes (genes that foster the growth and promotion of cancer) and up-regulate the expression of tumor suppressor genes.

When we eat, we're literally changing the expression of our genes, telling our cells which genes to turn on and which to silence! With every bite of food, meal after meal, day after day, cancer patients can leverage their power as "epigenetic engineers" to re-engineer their health.

It may turn out that our dinner fork is one of the most powerful anti-cancer tools we have in our toolbox!

Q: What foods and liquids might be considered helpful and what foods and liquids might be considered injurious or harmful?

A: Ah, people do like to have a definitive list of foods to avoid; we want a clearly identified enemy, a culinary culprit we can kibosh! And speaking very generally, there are some foods and beverages likely to be deleterious to nearly anyone who regularly partakes of them:

- Refined, processed and packaged foods with their excessive sugar
- GMOs and artificial ingredients
- Pesticide- or hormone-laden factory-farm-raised meats/poultry/dairy/eggs
- Preserved meats and fish with nitrates
- Soft drinks and alcoholic beverages
- Refined vegetable oils
- Hydrogenated and trans fats

But the real story is that any specific food or beverage might be unhealthy for one person, harmless or neutral for another, and possibly beneficial for yet another individual.

Breaking your fast each morning with a donut, bagel or bowl of "healthy" whole-grain cereal might be generally tolerable for an active individual with good blood sugar control, but harmful for someone with insulin resistance or gluten intolerance.

Steak for dinner? Perhaps beneficial during cancer treatment when one's protein requirement doubles and low protein status contributes to severe low blood counts that are sluggish to rebound. But regular meat intake is definitely worrisome for someone with hemochromatosis (excess iron stores). Char-grilling that same steak to well done? Carcinogenic compounds— heterocyclic amines (HCAs) and polyaromatic hydrocarbons (PAHs)—will be formed.

But people vary in their susceptibility. Many people inherit a slow-acting or more rapidly acting form of the N-acetyltransferase enzymes, NAT1 or NAT2, which modify susceptibility to developing cancer from these carcinogens. The underlying theme here is that there are many individual factors that exert their influence, so it's not truly possible to provide a set list of foods everyone needs to avoid.

For the foods to emphasize, it's the same story. Specific foods and beverages that are regularly reported in research studies to have anti-cancer effects include:

- Cruciferous vegetables (including broccoli, cabbage, cauliflower, kale, collards, Brussels sprouts, radish and mustard)
- Carotenoid-rich fruits and vegetables (known for their deep orange, red and yellow hues)
- Leafy greens
- Berries
- Spices
- Green tea

This "who's who" list of anti-cancer superstars, it turns out, are the very foods being shown to have epigenetic effects in modifying gene expression! Of course, there are individual factors at play here too, so it's not truly possible to provide a set list of foods everyone should eat.

Q: Regarding food, what does the term "glycemic load" mean and is the glycemic load of foods relevant to helping cancer patients?

A: When you eat carbohydrates, glucose is released into the blood stream. This is the fate of all carbs, be they simple or complex. In mainstream thinking, sweets and refined carbohydrates quickly release lots of glucose, whereas whole grains and complex carbohydrates release somewhat less glucose and do so at a slower pace, so they've been touted as healthier choices.

Glycemic Load (GL) and an earlier iteration called Glycemic Index (GI) are guides that were developed in order to quantify the relative blood-sugar elevating properties of foods. GI tells you how rapidly a particular carbohydrate turns into sugar. It doesn't tell you how much of that carbohydrate is in a serving of a particular food.

That's where GL comes in. Glycemic Load is a newer way to assess the impact of carbohydrate consumption that gives a fuller picture. It's calculated by multiplying a food's GI (as a percentage) by the number of net carbohydrates in a serving (that's total carbs minus fiber in grams).

Because it accounts for serving size and net carbs, glycemic load is considered a better indicator than glycemic index. For example, watermelon is high GI (76; where < 55 is considered low and > 70 is high), but since it contains few grams of carbohydrate, it's low GL (GL for a 1 cup serving is 3 where < 10 is low and > 20 is considered high).

There are some major failings in relying on glycemic load as a guide to shift our diets in a healthier direction.

First, it doesn't account for fructose or high-fructose corn syrup (HFCS). Our diets have morphed from supplying 16-20 grams/day, mostly from fresh fruits, to 85-100 grams of fructose per day, mostly from added HFCS now ubiquitous in packed foods and beverages. Fructose has a low GI and GL because, rather than raising blood glucose levels directly, it goes to the liver. High amounts of fructose in the liver readily stimulate the production of triglycerides and induce insulin resistance. So sodas and energy drinks sporting up to six grams fructose are listed as having a glycemic load of 0-1 (See www.nutritiondata.com.)

A second failing of glycemic load charts: They tell you about a food, but what about the characteristics of the person that influence glycemic response? Two people eating the same 1-cup serving of brown rice will not show the same glycemic response!

So it's likely no surprise when I state, in truth, we haven't found simply counting glycemic load points to be particularly helpful to the majority of our clients. Our finding is, and also that reported in a number of studies: Nearly every cancer patient tested—including non-diabetic patients—exhibits glucose intolerance, altered insulin secretion and insulin resistance. For these individuals, switching from high to low-glycemic load breads, cereals and pastas isn't enough. They need to greatly reduce their starch intake. This might mean eating a grain-free diet and getting all one's carbohydrates from vegetables, or possibly exploring a Ketogenic-type diet approach. The key here is watching the blood work indicators of insulin resistance, making diet changes, retesting, and repeating until we get the values in the target range.

And making these changes can be exceedingly important. Published reports link insulin resistance to poorer outcome in cancer patients, showing significantly increased rates of tumor recurrence and cancer spread.

The layperson's understanding has been that cancer cells are veritable Pac-Men gobbling up sugar. But the truth is more nuanced. Insulin resistance—when cells, having long faced a glut of dietary glucose, stop responding to insulin's request to stuff themselves with more of the sweet stuff—has metabolic effects that influence cancer via several mechanisms which, according to a study by Cowey and Hardy in 2006, include:

- Fueling inflammation, a well-established tumor promoter.
- Elevating insulin levels; insulin is directly mitogenic (promotes cell division of cancer cells).
- Promoting angiogenesis, the development of a dense network of new blood vessels, which supports tumor expansion.
- Increasing the secretion of leptin from fat cells (leptin is mitogenic, pro-angiogenic, and prompts cancer cell migration).
- Fostering unchecked free radicals, which increase DNA damage and contribute to genetic instability.
- Boosting circulating estrogen levels (Vona-Davis et al., 2007); (elevated estrogen is problematic in many types of cancer—independent of estrogen receptors on the surface of the cancer cells—because it can lead to high copper levels that foster angiogenesis).
- Suppressing immune function, our first line of defense against migrating cancer cells.

Q: How about specific diets? Many so-called cancer pundits push certain kinds of anti-cancer diets such as: gluten free, macrobiotic, ketogenic, paleo, raw, vegetarian or vegan, among others. What is your opinion about cancer diets?

A: Our approach is non-dogmatic. We don't believe any single diet approach is appropriate for everyone.

Consider this analogy, also drawn from my garden. Gardening in "raised beds"—the practice of growing crops in a bed of loosened soil mounded up above ground level—is widely touted as a beneficial strategy. But really, it depends. If you're in a wet or cool climate, have compacted soils or poor soil drainage, or wish to get an early jump on the season with a spring crop, raised beds can be advantageous. But in a desert climate—with its unrelenting sun, minimal rainfall and drying winds—a better strategy would be sunken beds, which help direct and conserve moisture. Similarly, it's ridiculous to suggest that any one diet is The Ideal Anti-Cancer Diet for everyone.

There are advantages and disadvantages to each of these diet approaches. While some of our clients might thrive on a vegetarian diet, others will be healthier eating some humanely raised, pasture-fed/finished meat. While a Gerson-type diet (organic plant-based) will provide ample phytonutrients for modifying gene expression, it can be disastrous to one's blood sugar control. Ditto macrobiotic approaches, which can be very healing for individuals whose genetic predisposition suits them to such an eating plan, but will worsen insulin resistance in others. A raw foods diet often works well as a short-term intervention to increase one's connectedness to food vibrancy, but carotenoids and other flavonoids have low bioavailability in their raw state and are optimized when cooked and eaten with healthy fats. The report we provide to our clients discusses all the major diet approaches and enumerates their benefits and potential drawbacks.

The question becomes: What effect does this specific diet plan have on my body? And then: Does it create an internal environment conducive to healing or one that favors cancer progression or recurrence? Are there important anti-cancer nutrients I'm likely to be deficient in with this eating plan (e.g., zinc, omega-3 fats, magnesium, CLA, etc.)?

It's paramount to tailor your diet to your unique biochemistry, metabolism, personal and cultural food preferences, allergies, and other factors. Our goal is to explain the benefits and drawbacks of the various approaches, so that you can capitalize on pearls of wisdom, take steps to overcome any potential drawbacks of the diet you choose for yourself, and merge all these considerations into a truly personalized "anti-cancer" diet. And that diet plan needs to be doable, delicious and rewarding—or you won't stick to it.

Q: How can someone ascertain what diet or nutritional approach may be best? Are there evidence-based tests, blood work or biochemical analyses that may be helpful to determine a best approach?

A: First and foremost, we check in with clients about how they are doing. How do they feel about the diet they're eating? Any changes in feelings of wellness and vitality? How's their digestion and elimination? Are there highs and lows in their energy level across the day? Any changes in symptoms or side effects, especially those known to be indicators of nutrient deficiency?

Another excellent tool we have for obtaining insight about one's diet is functional evaluation of blood chemistry (see Weatherby and Ferguson's *Blood Chemistry and CBC Analysis: Clinical Laboratory Testing from a Functional Perspective*). This little known area of functional medicine research can offer exciting feedback about how diet changes are impacting health and wellness.

Printed next to your results on the lab report, there's a column that defines an upper and lower limit called the reference range. Results outside this range help your doctor identify whether your state of health is so far deviated from normal, it's likely you have a medical condition that needs to be diagnosed and treated.

But if your result is within the range, does that mean you are optimally healthy? Not necessarily. Health is not merely the absence of disease! Let's take a closer look at what the reference range actually means, and decide if it is the standard against which you wish to compare yourself.

It would be ideal if individuals with superior health were studied in order to determine the optimal ranges for blood work results. Instead, reference ranges are determined statistically by collecting data from a large group of people who happen to be getting their blood tested, and then calculating the range within which 95 percent of that population falls. This method presupposes the population is healthy. But is it?

Studies on the incidence rates of various diseases report that 40-50 percent of individuals develop cardiovascular disease, 35 percent become diabetic, and 40 percent will be diagnosed with cancer in their lifetime. Alas, reference ranges reflect what is average, not what is optimal, for human health. So what target ranges do you want to use to help guide you in developing a nutrition and lifestyle plan to nourish your health?

When evaluating blood work from a nutritional perspective, you might wish to employ a narrower range: the optimal wellness range. For example, the lab reference range for potassium is 3.5-5.0 mmol/L. But for ideal health, many sources report a narrower range, 4.0-4.5 mmol/L, is optimal.

> **We've searched the published research to identify cut-off points on specific lab tests that are associated with optimal wellness, better prognosis, longer survival, or a reduced risk of cancer recurrence.**

The optimal target range helps define the specific environment within the body that is less hospitable to cancer growth and progression.

We teach clients how to decode their blood work results, so that as they make diet and lifestyle changes, they can ask, "How does my body respond when I am eating this way?" If a test result falls outside the target range, you can focus on dietary and lifestyle changes to help support it to return to the optimal range.

Q: Are your recommendations based upon the type of cancer and staging of that cancer, or are they based on other more personalized issues pertaining to a specific person's biochemistry?

A: Both!

Our guidance is always personalized. Tailoring a protocol to the unique needs and biochemistry of the individual is the foundation of our approach. But we also take into account numerous considerations relevant to the type and stage of cancer.

For example, many cancers—not just Estrogen Receptor Positive (ER+) breast cancer—are driven by estrogen, and this is a fertile arena to explore as many diet and lifestyle factors can influence estrogen pathways. Head and neck cancer, and gastric cancer patients have additional needs around a compromised ability to eat. Colorectal cancer clients, with portions of their intestines surgically removed, may have alterations in gut flora and reduced ability to absorb certain nutrients. Brain tumor protocols need to consider seizure risk and the ability of certain nutrients to cross the blood-brain barrier.

The list of contraindicated foods and supplements differs by type of cancer. All these considerations are added into the mix.

Q: What kinds of tests or blood work should a patient undertake and what should they be tested for?

A: One of the things that have fascinated me in the biomedical literature has been the exploration of biomarkers. Biomarkers are signs, or measurable parameters, associated with outcome. When a biomarker has been identified, it may be used to provide information on the likely course of the disease (prognostic biomarkers) or to identify subpopulations of patients most likely to respond to a given therapy (predictive biomarkers). The field of oncology predominately uses biomarkers to quantify risk, establish diagnosis, give treatment predictions or monitor response to treatment, and to predict likelihood of recurrence (such as the Oncotype DX breast cancer assay).

Most biomarkers are considered immutable characteristics of the disease, like stage at diagnosis, estrogen-receptor status, presence of invasion or metastasis, and key gene markers (p53, HER2, KRAS, EGFr, for example). But most intriguing to me are the many biomarkers that describe not the innate characteristics of the tumor cells, but the host terroir (what I've called the Oncometabolic Milieu). These are markers of systemic inflammation, insulin resistance, blood viscosity, angiogenic propensity, immune suppression, and nutrient imbalances (such as high copper, low zinc, or suboptimal vitamin D levels).

> These biomarkers are not static; they can be modulated
> by our diet and lifestyle choices. Our premise is that diet
> and lifestyle interventions to modify these biomarkers can
> give our clients the best odds of beating their prognosis, of
> surviving and thriving.

Each of these biomarkers has been associated in the literature with poorer prognosis or survival, increased risk of cancer spread or recurrence, and/or reduced treatment efficacy. This research is presented to our clients in their program materials.

A basic panel many of our clients run includes the following tests:

High-sensitivity (or cardio-) C-reactive protein, a measure of silent, systemic inflammation. For example, Professor Donald McMillan of the School of Medicine, University of Glasgow and his colleagues, measured C-reactive protein levels (inflammation status) in a group of 772 patients with lung, colorectal, gastric or breast cancer. They found low CRP was a strong, independent predictor of survival, and was an even better indicator of outcome than stage of disease (2001). Since this publication, more than 200 studies have also reported a strong association between inflammation, as measured by CRP, and prognosis, survival or recurrence rates across all types of cancers.

Glycated hemoglobin A1c as a lead indicator of insulin resistance. We're also interested to see additional indicators of insulin resistance on the blood work, such as fasting glucose, triglycerides, HDL cholesterol, uric acid, or fasting insulin levels.

Fibrinogen (activity) or D-dimer, as a marker of blood viscosity. Tumor cells can produce fibrin, a sticky, "clotty" protein, and appear to use it to hide from immune surveillance. Viscous blood may also impede the delivery of chemotherapy agents to their target sites and reduce treatment efficacy. And some studies suggest high fibrinogen correlates to increased risk of metastasis.

Vitamin D status (25-OH-cholecalciferol). There are several mechanisms of action by which vitamin D might impact cancer. It has been shown to induce differentiation (reversion of cancer cells to a more normal phenotype), promote apoptosis (programmed cell death), inhibit invasion, angiogenesis and metastasis, and help promote insulin sensitivity. In a recent study, for example, high serum vitamin D levels were associated with improved survival after a diagnosis of breast cancer (Mohr, et al., 2014).

Serum copper and ceruloplasmin (the copper binding protein). Elevated copper is one of the factors associated with angiogenesis, the growth of new blood vessels that supports tumor expansion. In fact, the key enzymes that drive angiogenesis require copper as a cofactor for their activation. Copper levels have been shown to rise during active disease and fall to normal during remission. Trials of copper chelation therapy have shown activity in stabilizing disease.

Depending on the type of cancer, it may also be useful to look at ferritin, lactate dehydrogenase (LDH), alkaline phosphatase (ALP), a thyroid panel (TSH, free T3 and free T4) and/or a comprehensive estrogen panel.

This simple panel of lab tests allows our clients to tailor their plan to their body's unique biochemical needs, prioritize which areas most need support, and set specific wellness goals. Retesting at intervals, say three and six months later, can help them gauge the efficacy of their nutrition protocol and make adjustments to their plan.

Q: Another controversial topic is supplementation. Vitamins, botanicals, herbs, extracts, and other agents that may be ingested or directed into the body have been questioned significantly recently. What is your opinion about different kinds of supplements?

A: We're not at all opposed to supplements when they are wisely chosen (based on rationale and testing), carefully screened for potential interactions or contraindications, and selected from companies that demonstrate a strong commitment to purity and potency in their manufacturing practices.

Meeting these criteria usually means you need to consult a nutrition professional with expertise working with cancer patients.

> **Having said this, we do very strongly feel that a healthy
> diet must form the foundation for any protocol.
> Supplements cannot replace a healthy diet with its thou-
> sands of phytonutrients and active constituents, many of
> which may yet remain to be discovered.**

Q: Just like pharmaceutical drugs, are the concepts of dosage, bioavailability (absorption), timing and the nature of specific brands of supplements important?

A: These considerations may be even more important with dietary supplements. For example, fat-soluble vitamins (such as carotenoids, and vitamins A, D, E and K) need to be taken with meals containing healthy fats in order to be absorbed. Some herbs have the same requirement, such as turmeric (the source of curcumin). Taking a supplement with or without food could potentially alter its effect. Bromelain, a proteolytic enzyme derived from pineapple, works as a digestive aid when taken with food, but demonstrates anti-inflammatory properties when taken between meals.

If reports by Consumer Labs are any indication, a significant proportion of over-the-counter brand supplements may not contain the amounts of ingredients listed on the label, or may contain contaminants. Our clients get access to our online resource guide that permits them to: 1) identify professional quality brands so they can select products produced under strict manufacturing standards and independently tested for purity, superior potency, and consistent quality; 2) learn when and how to take each supplement for best absorption, bio-availability, and maximum efficacy; and, 3) review the possible side effects, interactions, and contraindications for each agent.

Q: Should different patients with the same cancer take different kinds of supplements or the same kinds of supplements?

A: We've had clients with whom we are working meet each other online or at a conference and be stunned, upon comparing notes, that their diet and nutritional protocols are vastly different despite the fact that they share the same medical diagnosis!

Western medicine promotes the idea that treatments must be specific to the condition, but we favor the view that diet and nutrition must be individually tailored to the person.

> **One person with breast cancer may have high levels of inflammation and angiogenic markers, while another woman with the same type and stage of breast cancer may instead have insulin resistance and hormone imbalance. Giving these women the same 'breast cancer protocol' would be a disservice.**

Readers who'd like to explore this concept further can view our six-minute video presentation on the topic, on our home page (upper left hand corner) at our website: www.nutritional-solutions.net.

Q: Is there much laboratory or clinical evidence, including peer reviewed medical literature, supporting the purported efficacy of supplementation?

A: There are thousands of published studies on cancer and nutrition, studies on specialized diets, individual food items, proteins, fats, enzymes, vitamins, minerals, phytonutrients, herbs, lifestyle choices and more.

My Zotero database houses more than 8,750 studies I've read over the past 18 years. Each of these studies is like a single puzzle piece: as a stand alone, it doesn't amount to much. But when hundreds of these pieces are adeptly joined together, compelling patterns emerge and coherent ideas solidify. The bigger picture becomes clear.

Our Translational Research efforts involve three steps: 1) systematically and critically reviewing large volumes of research across multiple disciplines; 2) extrapolating and synthesizing that information into evidence-based protocols; and 3) fine-tuning those protocols based on continuous feedback from our clients.

The concept of evidence-based medicine is often trotted out, in regards to nutrition and complementary cancer therapies, to suggest that the only evidence worthy of our consideration comes from large scale, multi-institution, randomized, double-blind, placebo-controlled trials—the standard for evaluating drug treatments. But when the concept was first defined in the British Medical Journal in 1996, David Sackett wrote: "Evidence-based medicine is the conscientious, explicit, and judicious use of current best evidence in making decisions about the care of individual patients. The practice of evidence-based medicine means integrating individual clinical expertise with the best available external clinical evidence from systematic research."

Evidence-based medicine doesn't mean 'do nothing until more studies are done.' After all, when you have cancer, you need answers today.

Q: From where do you derive your research?

A: We predominately examine peer-reviewed studies in mainstream medical journals such as those available via PubMed. However, our clinical judgment often comes into play as well. For example, while there might not be any published research about potential side effects or interactions for a dietary supplement, if we've observed these kinds of effects or can make a rationale for potential harm, we don't hesitate to share the information with our clients.

Q: Why do you think so many doctors who treat cancer are against the concept that supplementation may be beneficial, specifically in helping create an inhospitable environment for cancer? Many doctors seem dogmatic in their opposition to this complementary option. Your thoughts?

A: Well, to go on record, I'd like to state emphatically that our office has NOT found the majority of oncologists with whom our clients work to be opposed to supplements.

Occasionally we do see this stance, and I think there are a few reasonable explanations. Foremost, ever since the discovery of penicillin, our culture has cultivated a mythos of the "magic bullet," the idea that we could develop a simple pill to cure each ill.

Since 1971, we've declared and literally waged a war on cancer, with aggressive, toxic, and expensive therapies to kill the rogue cells.

> **With this mindset, it's reasonable to question how some 'wimpy' foods or supplements could have any effect against our most formidable foe. Medical doctors are not trained in the science of how foods and nutrients contribute to health, and they have no tools in their toolbox for this job.**

There is truth in this saying: "If all you have in your toolbox is a hammer, every problem looks like a nail." This is why we believe partnering with oncologists is so essential, to give our clients the best of both worlds. Allopathic doctors may be wary due to concerns about interactions. As physicians have not received training about dietary supplements, they may take the stance of avoidance to protect their patients from potential interactions or side effects. When we partner with a doctor's office, we can provide in-depth information about the pharmacokinetics of dietary supplements. Our team has developed a cutting-edge, comprehensive model for screening interactions.

We take into consideration:

1) **Absorption:** Some foods and supplements can interfere with a drug's absorption (such as calcium, magnesium, and soluble fibers like psyllium, chia seed or flaxseed meal), reducing the intended efficacy of the drug. Other substances can increase absorption of various drugs (e.g., piperine from black pepper or bromelain, an enzyme in pineapples) leading to increased risk of side effects and possibly toxicity.

2) **Metabolism/Biotransformation:** Once the drug is absorbed, the liver has the job of metabolizing it, using a complex system of enzymes called the cytochrome p450. Some drugs depend upon these enzymes to be metabolized into their active form. Most drugs require CYP450 enzymes in order to be broken down and excreted from the body. The various enzymes are named in number-letter-number combinations, like 1A1, 1A2, 2D6, 3A4, and so on. A great majority of medications use the 3A4 pathway. Some foods (like grapefruit) and supplements also use this pathway, and herein is where the trouble begins. If they compete with each other, the drug might not be properly metabolized. Some substances up-regulate 3A4 (or other pathways) and can speed clearance of the drug, reducing its efficacy. Other substances can down-regulate 3A4, reducing the drug's metabolism or removal from the body, and lead to higher than intended blood levels of the drug, side effects, and toxicity.

3) **Individual polymorphisms (SNPs):** Just as our fingerprints are unique, so are the many genes that make up our CYP450, and changes in the make-up of these genes are called Single Nucleotide Polymorphisms (SNPs or "snips"). SNPs occur when a single "letter" (nucleotide) that makes up a "word" within a gene is substituted—say there's an A where a T should be, or a C replaces a G. The misspelling leads the enzyme to have an altered function. This can explain why some people have severe side effects or toxicity when taking a drug that is widely regarded as safe. If you have a SNP in a key CYP450 enzyme, a number of supplements may pose a risk to you, even though that supplement is generally considered to be safe and

benign. While testing for SNPs is expensive and not widely available, a client's history of previous drug reactions can provide clues as to SNPs they might carry. Innovative hospitals are beginning to apply pharmacogenetic testing to help physicians prescribe medicines more safely. St. Jude's has a pioneer program.

4) **Nutrient depletions:** Does the drug deplete any essential nutrients? Might these suboptimal nutrient levels increase risk of side effects and impact quality of life? The nutrient depleting effects of prescription drugs are widely overlooked, with the exception of the growing awareness that antibiotics deplete probiotics, the 100+ trillion bacteria comprising a healthy gut microbiome. Magnesium can be depleted by a wide variety of drugs, including antacids, acid blockers, antibiotics, blood pressure medications, diuretics, and corticosteroids. Estrogen-blocking drugs—the selective estrogen receptor modulators (SERMs, like Tamoxifen, Raloxifene and Toremifene) and the aromatase inhibitor Arimidex—also deplete magnesium. Combine these with a high-sugar diet, prolonged calcium supplementation, regular alcohol or coffee consumption, or malabsorption (as is common during and after chemotherapy) and magnesium wasting is exacerbated. Adequate magnesium is essential for good mood, relaxation, bone health, blood sugar balance, brain protection and inhibiting excess blood viscosity. Several drugs can deplete vitamin D, including: corticosteroids (decadron or prednisone often used as a chemo pre-med), laxatives, Dilantin and certain cholesterol-lowering drugs. Suboptimal levels of vitamin D could then reduce the efficacy of bone-strengthening drugs, like the bisphosphonates, and increase joint pain and osteonecrosis in those taking aromatase-inhibitors.

5) **Mechanism of actions:** Does the supplement work via a mechanism of action similar to the drug, perhaps competing for binding sites? For example, let's consider the anti-angiogenesis drug Avastin and its target receptor. Vascular endothelial growth factor (VEGF), is one factor that promotes angiogenesis (the growth of new tumor blood vessels), and Avastin blocks this process by binding to VEGF. A handful of botanical

agents, notably quercetin, resveratrol, St. John's wort and soy isoflavones have also been shown to have anti-VEGF effects. It's unknown whether combining any of these herbs with Avastin would prove synergistic, or whether the supplement might compete with the drug and reduce its efficacy. Two other botanical anti-VEGF agents, green tea and curcumin, on the other hand, do not bind to the VEGF binding site as Avastin does. These two herbs inhibit VEGF in different ways and might be compatible with the drug, perhaps even enhancing each other's anti-VEGF efforts (though curcumin in high doses could increase bleed risk associated with Avastin).

6) **Side effect amplification:** If a drug is likely to cause diarrhea, caution should be used with any supplements that may exacerbate that risk, such as high doses of fish oil, magnesium or vitamin C. Does the drug carry a risk of heightened photosensitivity reactions? If so, herbs like St. John's wort, fennel, angelica, and lomatium may need to be avoided. If a drug causes blood thinning, a long list of supplements needs to be considered as risky, including the "4G"s: ginkgo, garlic, ginger, and ginseng. This bleed risk would be magnified in a client who had a low platelet count, and perhaps minimized in one with a recent history of clots, elevated fibrinogen or other markers of blood viscosity. So personalized risk assessment, on a case-by-case basis, is needed.

Now that you've had a chance to learn more about the complexities, you can see the limited usefulness of online pharmacy databases to declare a list of supplements definitively contraindicated. We believe that screening for interactions needs to be done on a case-by-case basis by a team of health care providers that includes advisors who are well versed in dietary supplements and nutritional medicine.

Q: How about studies? There are millions of studies globally in the medical literature today with polarized and partisan camps vehemently asserting that their viewpoint is correct and proven. We are bombarded weekly with reports of these studies in the media asserting that there is

a breakthrough drug to fight cancer or that a particular natural agent's benefits are unsubstantiated or, in the opposite case, quite efficacious.

A: This question could be the topic for an entire book. It's a pet peeve of mine! I'm known for exclaiming a long drawn out, "Whaaaaat?" and continuing in a mock voice, "Another poorly designed study on 'nutrient X' and cancer? Why didn't they consult me before wasting millions of dollars on this?"

But seriously, the National Institutes of Health (NIH) has put significant funding into research on nutrition and cancer, and that's a good thing. Sadly, it's my observation that many of the investigators getting these grants do not know enough about nutrition to do meaningful, well-designed studies.

In addition, they're using a research model that was developed for drug research, and it's just not appropriate or adequate for evaluating the impact of nutrition. For example, in a drug study, you give each subject the same dose (adjusted by body weight). In nutrient studies, each subject comes into the study with a different baseline level of the nutrient, varying rates of absorption, different levels of co-factors and synergists, diverse intake—see where I'm heading?

Giving each participant the same 400 IU dose of vitamin E or 200 mcg of selenium, for example, is fraught with error. Even if you measure blood levels of the nutrient, you can still miss the mark since biochemical individuality data has shown that the levels of a nutrient needed to achieve the same biological outcome can vary 20 to 200-fold across individuals. Perhaps my immune cells are fortified against infection with 60 mg vitamin C, while yours need 1,200 mg to be similarly bolstered.

An equivalent blood level of an antioxidant nutrient may be ideal for one participant, yet barely begin to scratch the surface of excessive oxidation in another. And, in a third, that dose could prove excessive and cause immune suppression and interfere with necessary oxidation needed to burn calories and produce energy.

Moreover, the realization of synergistic interdependence of nutrients is overlooked and is a significant confounding variable in studies. Giving high doses of any nutrient can cause functional deficiencies of other nutrients. For example, vitamin D is part of a network of fat-soluble vitamins including vitamin K2 and vitamin A. Taking high doses of vitamin D can cause functional deficits of the others. So then, when it comes time to draw conclusions about a study's null or negative finding, you have to wonder—is this nutrient actually causing harm or did they really just measure the effect of *depleting* vitamins K2 and A? Ditto for studies on alpha tocopherol, often mistakenly treated as "vitamin E" though it's only one of the eight compounds comprising the vitamin E family. Taking isolated alpha tocopherol depletes the other tocopherols and tocotrienols which seem to be the true anti-cancer powerhouses.

Consider the widely fluctuating reports about calcium and the risk of bone fractures: "it helps" versus "is no help at all" versus "is potentially harmful, increasing cardiovascular disease risk." Well, bone health is like a complex recipe for a cake. You can't bake a cake with flour alone, or eggs alone. Even when you've got all the necessary ingredients sitting on the counter, you still need to carefully measure out the correct amounts, because 2 cups of baking soda and 1 teaspoon almond flour do not make it delicious. Ditto bones: You need all the ingredients in the correct amounts: calcium, vitamin D, vitamin K2, magnesium, boron, and maybe strontium.

But we have a research model that says, test one variable at a time to see if A causes B. So if a study on calcium alone, or vitamin D alone, or even calcium plus D fails to find a significant effect, what does that tell us? Perhaps in Study #1, calcium was no help because the study participants were deficient in vitamins D and K2, whereas in Study #2, calcium was found to be effective because the participants had good levels of the supportive network of nutrients.

Likewise, all the conflicting reports on "antioxidants"? Guess what? It's a very complex cake recipe with a network of ingredients working synergistically to maintain a dynamic balance between oxidation and reduction. It's not about how one nutrient quenches all the oxidation. So what does a study about a single nutrient, say vitamin E, tell us about antioxidants? Not much.

Many nutrition studies are epidemiological in nature. The diet or habits of a population are explored to discern associations between health outcomes—say cancer risk, and certain foods, nutrients or diet patterns. What's often overlooked when these studies are reported in the media is that their findings show correlation, not causation: "A" is associated with "B," not "A" causes "B." It's quite plausible that an unmeasured third factor is the key.

Do some studies show a correlation between red meat intake and cancer because, in our culture, meat eaters are more likely to smoke, drink alcohol, fail to eat adequate amounts of protective foods like vegetables, or engage in other habits that increase cancer risk? Is it perhaps not the meat itself, so much as the method of cooking or nitrates added to preserved meats like bacon and hot dogs? Or maybe it's the poor ratio of omega-6 to omega-3 fatty acids in factory-farm-raised meats that explain the observed risk.

It's a reminder not to take reports of these studies at face value. I generally find such studies generate far more questions than they answer!

Q: Should we scrutinize these studies carefully? In other words, do we need to question the financial sponsors, the design of the studies, the scientists, the nature of the drugs or natural agents, and investigate myriad other factors?

A: Yes, we do need to scrutinize studies carefully and examine all the factors you mention. Often the in-depth and behind-the-scenes knowledge to do this kind of analysis are out of the reach of the lay public. We've found this simple dictate can be helpful in navigating the contradictory and ever-changing headlines: Never draw conclusions on the basis of a single study. You see, cancer research is like the parable of the blind men exploring an elephant, each having taken hold of a different body part. Any single study is merely the finding of one narrow perspective. We need to put all the data pieces together in order to see clearly the state of understanding as it currently stands (this evolves over time). This is the value of Translational Research and clinical experience.

So when the next wild, attention-grabbing, contradictory headline wends its way into the public eye, you can begin to ask some judicious questions. What do other studies on this topic say? (You can search PubMed free at www.ncbi. nlm.nih.gov.) How does this study differ from other studies on this same topic? Are there alternate explanations for the finding? Were important confounding factors identified? What was the form, dose, duration and delivery method of the nutrient? Did they use a clinically relevant dose? Was it given for long enough to produce a measurable effect? Did they use appropriate means of measuring the outcome?

Q: Can we patently trust the results or does the potential for bias, driven by financial and other issues compromise results from time to time? I believe uninformed people and, in fact, the medical community itself, can become confused by media sound bites taken from the results of scientific papers and the plethora of studies. Your thoughts?

A: Reports that have catalogued the incidence of bias, misreporting, method-ological errors, and other compromises do reveal a high frequency of problems in the biomedical literature. It's a serious concern.

It's particularly disconcerting when uninformed or confused reports go uncorrected. It's not uncommon for a later analysis or follow-up studies to discover significant flaws in a highly publicized study. Or a re-analysis of the data may discover the finding is limited to a specific subgroup of individuals. Corrections and clarifications rarely make headlines, so erroneous information is still floating around.

I think many of us are beginning to ignore these constant media-sensation-alized reports. There's the impression that the boy has cried wolf too often.

Frankly, our team is on a mission. We're busy serving our clients, and it is draining to have to be pulled away from that work to address yet another poorly done study, misrepresentation or wild claim. We've started teaching our clients and Facebook community how to evaluate research studies, so they can see the wizard behind the curtain for themselves. Denise Minger's book *Death by Food Pyramid* has a lovely chapter on these skills, and Tom Naughton has a hilarious and highly informative video on YouTube called "Science for Smart People" that teaches critical appraisal skills.

Do all these problems mean we should just throw out all the millions of studies cramming the cyber-shelves at the National Library of Medicine? Not at all. It means we need to ask probing questions, proceed with critical appraisal, and then vet the findings in our personal lives and with individual clients. It means we need to value and seek out those experts in the field who can use their expertise to critically evaluate the studies.

You wouldn't ask your car mechanic to perform your next root canal, nor rely on your neurosurgeon to install the electrical system in your new home. Isn't it odd that many people expect the services of a specialist to be able to handle the job that needs to be done, but are willing to take nutritional guidance from anyone?

Even when a study is impeccably well designed, conducted and appropriately analyzed, we still should not blindly trust the outcome. Published nutrition studies should be used as a jumping off point, as a general guideline for where to get started. Each client needs to vet the information for his/her particular situation and body chemistry.

For instance, say that you're eating a vegetarian diet, but when you test your oncometabolic markers they're far from the target ranges. You switch your diet plan around, reduce your starch intake, maybe add some wild-caught cold-water fish, more healthy fats, and those same indicators move into range. You've just discovered Your Personal Anticancer Diet, and it doesn't matter what the conflicting studies assert.

Q: Can you outline how you and your colleagues go about your "personal consultation" process with new patients?

A: The process begins before a person becomes a client. Our office manager and client coordinator have conversations with prospective clients and with new clients going through the intake process by phone, email, and sometimes Skype. This is in order for us to better understand each client's interests, concerns and resources. It also serves in helping each client to better understand how he or she can prepare for his or her first consultation, to make it as effective and efficient as possible. If it would be useful to review certain reading material or acquire certain tests prior to consulting with us, this is a time when that comes to light.

Helping each client increase his or her cancer nutrition knowledge base is our first goal. Each program we offer comes with one of my signature translational research reports specific to the diagnosis or treatment the client is facing. You might say these reports are the mature fruit of my ongoing translational research in cancer nutrition. They have been my life's work since 1996, reviewing more than 8,750 studies and counting. With this comprehensive text, clients begin to narrow down the pool of information to consider, from cancer nutrition in general to brain tumor nutrition, ovarian cancer nutrition, melanoma nutrition, or nutrition during radiation, for example.

Clients receive their program packet ahead of their first consultation. In addition to the report, this packet contains a set of quick reference guides and worksheets developed as a companion to the reports. The quick reference sheets offer dietary inspiration and direction, as well as ways to put the dietary principles into action. They begin the transition from translational cancer research to the kitchen. The worksheets have evolved out of our clinical experience fostering in others a deep personal understanding of cancer nutrition as a manner of living. These program materials function as a reference text and workbook from which our clients build their diet, supplement, and lifestyle practices.

But of course, clients don't do that alone. Not by a long shot! I'm fortunate to be working with one the world's most uniquely qualified cancer nutrition clinicians, Michelle Gerencser, M.S., who readily innovates nutrition protocols and our incomparable consulting method on an ongoing basis, one client at a time. Michelle takes each clients hand and wisely guides him or her through the process of applying the translational research in daily life, deciding what's the focus, and prioritizing what is clinically relevant for each individual.

Michelle teaches our clients how to make nutritional decisions using personal facts and careful analysis. This places the research in a personal context. Data such as lab tests, at-home testing, metabolic measurements, and symptoms uncover therapeutic opportunities. This part of personalizing the consultation manifests as a methodical discussion of a diet self-evaluation worksheet, blood work log, current symptoms, and perhaps other test results. The goal of the discussion is to identify the oncometabolic factors and other concerns that are of highest priority for that individual at that time.

Phone or Skype consultations also allow for intangible preferences and concerns to come to light and be figured in as the analysis becomes more and more personal. In this way, decision-making is collaborative. The process is actually quite orderly for all that is taken into account. It is informed by facts, and supported by rigorous analysis. It's also subject to constant re-analysis and re-interpretation over time.

The Nutrition Planner, a protocol sheet developed for each client during his/her phone consultation, provides a tangible conclusion and a jumping off place for action. This spreadsheet documents a client's nutritional plans, rationales for those plans, and timing for follow-up monitoring. It summarizes intentions and provides a detailed action plan in a short format.

Email consultations are often used between phone consultations to solidify knowledge, hone implementation of the nutrition plan, and build confidence in applying the new information. We even have a hotline for clients who need immediate assistance with treatment-related side effects.

Q: Are there any types of cancer patients whom you will not work with, or are you open to most types of cancer issues?

A: Our team offers our consulting services for clients with all types of cancer. We work with clients throughout their care, from support during cancer treatments to post-treatment recovery and assistance, and reducing the risk of reccurence thereafter.

Sometimes our philosophy and goals are not a match for what a potential client is seeking. Our relationship with our clients is educational rather than prescriptive. Our clients enjoy taking an active role in developing their nutritional approaches. Their desire is to build a strong anti-cancer environment within the body. They want to be educated about the rationale and level of research support available so that they can make informed decisions for themselves about diet, nutrition, and lifestyle approaches.

If someone is looking for a practitioner who will issue a "prescription" for a specific diet plan or supplements, or if they are looking for alternative treatments to directly kill cancer cells, those needs will be better served by a holistic medical practitioner.

Q: What is your vision, five or 10 years down the road, regarding the progress of cancer care?

A: My vision encompasses several themes. I'd like to see future approaches to cancer care that are less toxic, more personalized, holistic, and empowering.

1) **Less toxic:** I think it's time to stop waging war against cancer. Perhaps there is a kinder, gentler way? Our grand scheme of decimating the cells with toxic agents has been a dismal failure. It's time for a new approach. Perhaps our hypothesis that cancer cells are enemies resulting from DNA mutations is incorrect, and rather, as professors Carlos Sonnenchein and Anna Soto posit in their book *The Society of Cells*, the problem originates within the network of communications between cells and their environment, signals that function to organize and constrain cell behavior. Research emanating from this model may help us pave the way to innovative and non-toxic therapies aimed at restoring the body's healthy ecosystem.

2) **Personalized:** If a clinical trial examining a cancer drug (or natural agent) reported that the disease progressed in 90 percent of patients taking the drug, the agent would likely be deemed a failure and would be discarded as ineffective. But wait— what are the characteristics of those 10 percent whom the drug helped? Were they individuals with a certain

gene expression pattern? People who also took Metformin? Those with robust hemoglobin levels, elevated fibrinogen, or low folate levels? We have the computer technology for these kinds of sophisticated analyses; we just need to collect the data, and ask these types of questions. If we were able to pre-screen for those characteristics and re-test the drug only in these pre-selected individuals, it might help nearly all of them. If we're to increase our efficacy in helping people with cancer, it's imperative we begin to tailor all therapies—both conventional treatments and integrative approaches—to the individual. We need to stop thinking of people as machines: put 'x' in, get 'y' out.

3) **Patient-centered and holistic:** Medicine has been so narrowly focused on the tumor, that it's not uncommon for our clients to report to us that they feel like their medical team failed to see them, the whole person. Or a client will report their medical team is so focused on "the cancer," they have no interest in addressing the patient's depression, ongoing GI discomfort, cognitive changes (like "chemo brain"), or insomnia. More than a few clients have exclaimed, "What good is shrinking the tumor, if it doesn't extend my survival and ruins my quality of life for the time I have left?" We need to care for the whole person, and I dearly hope the field matures to tackle this deficiency.

4) **Empowered:** Increasingly savvy cancer patients are seeding a revolution: They want their power back and deserve to be full partners in directing their care. Indeed, their daily self-care has immense measurable healing results. We now have the opportunity to partner with them and turn the tide on our current rising tsunami of cancer incidence and mortality.

If you're reading this as a cancer survivor/thriver, welcome to the team. If you're feeling inundated with overwhelming stress, find a healthcare practitioner whom you can trust to steer the course until you're ready to take the wheel.

Q: Do you have any suggestions, or recommendations for people who were recently given a serious cancer diagnosis or experienced a serious

**recurrence issue, concerning how to handle heightened emotions—
and an appropriate approach to making critically important treatment
decisions?**

A: Breathe! Sigh! Let it be OK that there are at first, chaos, anxiety, concern and a sense of being overwhelmed.

These are reasonable responses to a cancer diagnosis or news of a recurrence. So let it be OK that your world feels turned upside down when you first get the news.

I'm inspired by a Buddhist concept that suffering arises in direct proportion to our struggle. If we try to plant our feet and resist the flow, the river rages against us; but if we lean back and float, we're at peace again.

Ever been white-water rafting? Skilled river guides give this advice about falling overboard and being sucked into turbulent waters: Curl up into a fetal position, trust that your personal floatation device will protect you, and let the river spit you out. Do not fight the current.

A cancer diagnosis is one of those times when we find ourselves unexpectedly tossed from the vessel and immersed in the turbulent waters. We can choose to struggle and exhaust our resources, or we can choose to let go, relax, breathe calmly and deeply, and simply allow the waters to support and carry us. Don't let cancer take over your entire life. A wise woman with invasive bladder cancer—my mom—shared with our Facebook community her unique strategy for effectively managing the stress:

> **"I am only going to have cancer before noon.
> It is too exhausting to be a cancer patient all day.
> Therefore, all cancer business must be accomplished
> before noon, and will have to be squeezed in
> before or after my hike."**

Devising a boundary so that you can focus on the enjoyable and nourishing parts of your life can be very healing, as can spending time outdoors in nature.

Our team strongly believes that treatment decisions need to honor the philosophy, beliefs and needs of the individual. There's no question the mind-body connection is a powerful healing force. To harness that power, align your thoughts and beliefs with your selected treatments. No one wants to be sitting in a treatment chair while doubting thoughts course through the mind.

Take time to investigate your options. Ask questions so you can be an informed consumer of the medical therapies you choose to undergo.

You can find our list of "Questions To Ask Your Doctor" online on Facebook at www.NutritionalSolutions/notes.

Don't be afraid to get a second, third, fourth and even fifth opinion regarding your treatment options! When Italian artist and engineer Salvatore Iaconesi was diagnosed with a brain tumor in September 2012, he hacked into his proprietary medical records, posted them online and crowd-sourced treatment options, asking the world to help him find a cure. In the space of a few weeks, hundreds of treatment suggestions came pouring in, ranging from evidence-based and complementary treatments to unconventional approaches involving poetry, art and music. While I applaud his resourcefulness, I wonder how he was able to weed through the options and select those best suited to him.

My advice? Expand your options, and have a plan for evaluating them. If you have knowledge of your Oncometabolic Milieu, you have a compass you can use to help navigate your way and prioritize your options.

References, Resources, and Attributions
from Jeanne Wallace, Ph.D., C.N.C.

1) Cowey, S., & Hardy, R. W. (2006). The Metabolic Syndrome. *The American Journal of Pathology, 169*(5), 1505-1522.

2) Mcmillan, D. C., Elahi, M. M., Sattar, N., Angerson, W. J., Johnstone, J., & Mcardle, C. S. (2001). Measurement of the Systemic Inflammatory

Response Predicts Cancer-Specific and Non-Cancer Survival in Patients With Cancer. *Nutrition and Cancer, 41*(1-2), 64-69.

3) Mohr, S.B., Gorham E.D., Kim, J., Hofflich, H., & Garland C.F. (2014). Meta-analysis of Vitamin D Sufficiency for Improving Survival of Patients with Breast Cancer. *Anticancer Research 34*(3), 1163–1166.

4) Vona-Davis, L., Howard-Mcnatt, M., & Rose, D. P. (2007). Adiposity, type 2 diabetes and the metabolic syndrome in breast cancer. *Obesity Reviews, 8*(5), 395-408.

ROBERT NAGOURNEY, M.D.

ABOUT ROBERT NAGOURNEY, M.D. Dr. Robert Nagourney is the medical and laboratory director at Rational Therapeutics. He is internationally known for pioneering the use of "functional profiling." He is a clinical professor of gynecologic oncology at the University of California, Irvine School of Medicine, and is board certified in internal medicine, medical oncology, and hematology.

At Boston University, Dr. Nagourney earned a B.A. in Chemistry, summa cum laude, Phi Beta Kappa with distinction in biochemistry. He received his medical degree at McGill University in Montreal, where he was a University Scholar. After completing his residency in Internal Medicine at the University of California, Irvine, he received fellowship training in medical oncology at Georgetown University in Washington, D.C. and went on to complete a second fellowship in hematology at the Scripps Institute in La Jolla, California, where he was the recipient of the Scripps Institute Young Investigator Award.

In 1993, Dr. Nagourney founded Rational Therapeutics where he pioneered the use of "functional profiling" to create the world's first personalized cancer therapy program. Two fundamental breakthroughs underlie the success of his approach. The first was the recognition that cancer reflected a deregulation of cell survival, not cell proliferation. The second reflected an understanding of cancer biology as cancer ecology, wherein cancer cells must be studied in their native state, not propagated, sub-cultured nor removed from their stroma, inflammatory and vascular environment.

With more than 20 years of experience in human tumor primary culture analyses, Dr. Nagourney has authored more than 100 manuscripts, book chapters, and abstracts, including publications in the Journal of Clinical Oncology, Gynecological Oncology and The Journal of National Cancer Institute. As co-investigator on national cooperative trials, he is recognized for the introduction of cisplatin/ Gemcitabine doublets in the treatment of advanced ovarian and breast cancers.

Dr. Nagourney is a frequently invited lecturer at numerous professional organizations and universities, and has served as a reviewer and on the editorial boards of several journals including Clinical Cancer Research, British Journal of Cancer, Gynecologic Oncology, Cancer Research and The Journal of Medicinal Food.

In 2013, Dr. Nagourney wrote Outliving Cancer (Basic Health Publications), about the discovery of the biology of cancer and how best to treat it.

Interview

Q. What life events or issues impelled you to become an oncologist?

A: It was almost by accident; I did not originally plan to pursue oncology. My interest was originally in biochemistry. It was recommended that I should meet with a fellow who was doing pharmacology research relating to cancer. I agreed to meet with him and he immediately struck me as a smart and capable guy.

I started working in his laboratory from that moment forward. Over the course of a couple years, I published two prestigious, peer-reviewed publications under his tutelage, launching me into the cancer arena. I felt it was an area of great need so I figured I would remain in a field that had a lot of tough issues, and that was cancer.

Q. Has the fight to inhibit or control advanced cancers improved much in the past few decades?

A: I think we are beginning to control cancers "around the edges." What I mean is, some of the "worst cancers" turn out to become the "best cancers."

For example, there was a very aggressive form of leukemia called promyelocytic leukemia, which was an absolutely lethal diagnosis. It was one of those diseases for which no one had any solutions. Lo and behold, someone discovered that this form of leukemia was driven by a retinoid receptor mutation. They showed that if you gave patients trans retinoic acid, they would go into remission. Thus, the "worst" form of leukemia became the "best," in terms of treatability.

Similarly, chronic myelogenous leukemia, which was also uniformly fatal, requiring a bone marrow transplant, became the target of a small molecule, STI- 571, known as Gleevec and that has revolutionized the management of this problem. Those kinds of advances, however, are only nibbling at the edges of cancer.

> **We are still not curing colon, recurrent breast, lung, pancreatic, recurrent ovarian, melanoma, gastric or other common cancers. We are doing a little better, but we are not having a big impact on the leading causes of cancer death.**

I feel more optimistic now than I did five or 10 years ago, but it will be a long, slow battle to make real progress with the common cancers.

Q. Are we not allocating enough resources to fight cancer?

A: We certainly spend a lot of money on cancer. One of the problems is that scientific research is a "herd mentality." People tend to go down the currently popular path. For the past 20 years, we have been engaged in the study of genomics and signal transduction. I think we will soon be confronted by the reality that evolution occurs at every level.

> **As you block one pathway, a new one will emerge and as you block that, a third pathway will supervene your inhibition. We are chasing 'leads,' but they are not cures. They give us brief remissions, followed by resistance.**

Some of the resistance phenomena that we encounter are even more aggressive than the diseases that we encountered in the first place. In terms of one of the big benchmarks, prolonging five-year survival, we are not having any impact—none whatsoever.

I am a great believer in fundamental biochemistry. In the long run, all of the molecular biology, which is what is funded by everyone today, will eventually lead us back to the more important areas like enzymology, bioenergetics, and cancer metabolism.

Q: Are the studies and trials erroneously designed or are the approaches flawed in these studies?

A: For two decades, I have been espousing the concept that patients should be treated based upon their own unique biology. Patients shouldn't get standardized treatments.

> **It is interesting to see that during the past five to 10 years everyone has awoken to 'individualized' or 'personalized' cancer treatments, but that they are only willing to 'personalize' treatment based upon genomic analyses, to the exclusion of other highly validated platforms.**

We use a platform that measures the biological response of cancer cells, a systems approach to tissue biology that has not yet been accepted by many scientists. While they desperately want to do what we are doing every day, their tunnel vision prevents them from applying the single most accurate and validated platform—functional analyses—to select treatments. They myopically adhere to genomic platforms, that at best can provide only a veneer of the information they so desperately desire, e.g. patient responsiveness to therapy.

Today's trials are increasingly focused on biomarkers. The trouble is that we only have a handful of biomarkers, yet there are millions of cancer patients who need help every year. It follows that not every patient fits a biomarker. Thus, they end up in the standardized treatment protocols, which are so distasteful from the standpoint of those who need to be treated, compared to those who actually respond (on average one in seven).

I am not happy with the clinical trial process.
It is very inefficient, costly and cumbersome.

Q. In addition to being a practicing oncologist with your own patients, you are well known as a physician who looks at cancer differently from most oncologists. What events or issues caused you to look at cancer differently from other doctors and scientists? Was there an "aha" moment or set of events that changed your perception?

A: I was working in a laboratory where we were developing small molecules. We were testing them in animals. Some of the work we were engaged in was going on to clinical trials, but they were not working very well. A lot of time, energy, and money went into these endeavors, despite the fact that they were not going well.

I subsequently met an investigator who was engaged in the study of human tumor primary culture studies. I thought, "Gee, wouldn't it be a better way to go?" If it were not for the fact that these tissue culture systems worked, I would have been only too happy to get out of the field, but right off the bat I began to see meaningful improvements in my patients' outcomes. In fact, I wrote my first abstract almost 30 years ago and presented it at the ASCO meeting in Toronto, regarding patients with leukemia who had previously failed therapy, but responded after I selected the drugs via the laboratory analysis.

I thought, however naively, "Now that I have shown that this works, people will rethink their naysaying and come around to my way of thinking." But that didn't happen. For years, I tried to figure out why people did not want to accept what we were doing. They did not want to accept increasingly good data.

In 1992, almost 10 years later, I heard the first formal description of the process of apoptosis and programmed cell death. I realized what I had been doing for the prior decade was measuring programmed cell death. I realized there was now a very credible, defensible scientific rationale for the merit of my work. Recognizing that it worked, with this newfound evidence, I was sure that this would be a turning point. But, the academics were so convinced that human tissue could not predict human outcome, that it did not matter how good the data was, nor how good the science or statistics were. In truth, scientists are very closed minded to many things, particularly those things that undermine or disrupt their belief systems.

Once you have a cadre of investigators who are convinced that human tissue cannot predict outcome, it does not matter if you cure every patient in the world; they will still say, dogmatically, that it does not work.

Q: Is today's essential paradigm that many oncologists and cancer centers use "off the shelf" chemotherapeutic drugs or protocols to attack or debulk tumors based on the name and stage of that cancer, versus customized, personalized approaches as you do?

A: The standard of care around the world today is disease type, stage and National Comprehensive Cancer Network (NCCN) guideline approaches.

You go to a doctor. They figure out the type of cancer you have. Then they stage you and finally they look at a book to decide on a treatment plan. That is 90 percent of cancer care today. Some small groups are offering genomic profiles, but unless you have a discrete mutation—and there are only a handful of patients who do—everything else is generic therapy.

> **We have the ability to not only measure whether chemo-therapy drugs work, but also to determine how the targeted agents work. The functional platform, the tissue culture platform, and the systems based platform is demonstrably better, but is still not widely applied.**

Q: What does the acronym "EVA-PCD" stand for and what does it mean? Your website speaks to this proprietary platform.

A: EVA is Ex Vivo Analysis, meaning removed from the body and analyzed; PCD is the measurement of drug-induced Programmed Cell Death.

For the most part, drugs that work in patients have an impact on cellular survival. Most cancer responses are injuries to the cancer cell's survival systems. One way or another, those treatments that work do so by leading to the death of the tumor as a whole. We have developed a platform, designed to measure how cell death is associated with growth factor withdrawal, or signal transduction inhibition, or cytotoxic insult, or radiation damage as it relates to tumor volume in the patient.

Ex Vivo Analysis means "out of body analysis." Programmed Cell Death is conducted by using these molecules, in short term culture, and measuring programmed cell death.

Q: Why have oncologists and other doctors been slow to accept functional profiling versus other testing methodologies? It would seem you cannot get more "personalized" in testing the efficacy of specific chemo drugs and combinations than with the actual patient's tissue sample. Are there historical reasons why acceptance has been slow, pertaining to current attitudes?

A: Since 1954 (Black and Spear, *Journal of the National Cancer Institute*, 1954), people have been trying to develop ways to predict chemotherapy response in the laboratory. The fact is that the results reported in that paper were positive. The investigators did in fact pick the winners and losers, but the reality was that there were only five drugs at the time. No one really cared. There was no need to pick them; you could easily treat patients with all the available drugs.

Years of drug development during the 1970s and 1980s led to dozens of new drugs. Now it became increasingly important to select the appropriate drug or combination of drugs.

Unfortunately, the preeminent belief at the time was that cancer was a disease of cell proliferation and unbridled growth. Since the middle of the 19th century, cancer had been viewed as a disease of cell growth, unregulated DNA synthesis followed by mitosis. Everyone assumed that the drug testing process would, per force of necessity, need to measure drug inhibition of cell growth.

It was that error that led the clonogenic assay, and the entities that offered these types of assays, to study cell growth. But it turns out that cancer is driven by survival factors, and that growth inhibition is irrelevant. These investigators and their investors found out that these assays did not predict anything. So instead of saying, "Maybe we should go back and rethink this," they concluded, erroneously, that this could never be done.

It would be as if someone said prior to the Wright Brothers, that heavier-than-air flight will never occur. It would be as if someone said to Steve Jobs, no one will ever develop a desktop computer that anyone would ever want to use. It would be as if someone said, before the existence of FedEx, that a private delivery service could never compete with the Post Office.

All of these attitudes are now in retrospect patently ridiculous. We are up against people who are dogmatic about their unwillingness to see the truth, while we have provided excellent data over the last two decades.

Q: How can we get doctors' attitudes to change so patients may receive the advantages of the most cutting-edge tests to ascertain which chemo drugs may be most beneficial, like functional profiling?

A: I thought this could be achieved by conducting clinical trials. Indeed, I spent about 10 years conducting and reporting the results of clinical trials. I took compounds and drug combinations that I developed in my laboratory, gave them to patients, and proved that they worked. Then I gave patients the combinations and did blinded correlations to show that the people that responded were those selected in the laboratory.

> **I gave people with advanced disease, drug combinations that I recommended and compared the results with the best outcomes provided by the very same naysayers. On each occasion, we improved the outcomes. I doubled the response rate and nearly doubled the survival in advanced non-small cell lung cancer. Yet, it has had no impact (on the mindset of the mainstream).**

Q: What is genomic profiling? Is that the same as molecular profiling?

A: We have come to define genomic analyses as molecular biology. In fact, it is a misnomer to use such a big term for such a limited scope of analyses.

What we are really talking about is genotypic analysis. In essence, your parents provide you with a set of genes. After a rather complicated set of unpredictable events, those genes become configured into what we call "you"— known as your phenotype.

A genotype is a "starting point" for what ultimately becomes "you." The problem with genetic analysis is that the genes are only a starting point of your biology. If you try to make a genotype into a person there is a high likelihood that a lot of the expression, proteins and interactive systems that make you "you" cannot be accurately described just from reading the "blueprint." What I say to people is, a blueprint can be turned around and read backwards and the building will look entirely different from what the original design was, even though it was read just as the blueprint specified.

It is overly simplistic to assume that your genotype is "you." It is not.

However, your phenotype is absolutely "you" and your cancer phenotype is the biology and behavior of your cancer cell, so we measure phenotype. I think this is a much better approximation of human biology. Phenotype is how the cell or the organ reads the genetic information, escapes the impact of small interfering RNAs, avoids the impact of pseudo-gene MRNAs, gets through the protein kinetics and configures whatever the information at the baseline is, and arrives at the finish line that defines your individual biology.

The finish line, your cellular behavior, then interacts with its vasculature and its microenvironment. The tissue culture systems that we use assess phenotypic biology within the microenvironment. The microenvironment is the interactive system of vasculature, inflammatory cells, stromal cells, and the cell-to-cell communication.

Genotype is a term for the starting point of genetic information; phenotype is a term for the biological product of genes.

Q: What would be the argument for someone who is a proponent of genomic testing, and in your opinion, why is it inadequate??

A: As the genotype is the starting point of your biology, the genomic investigator would say, "All biology is ultimately driven by genetic information." That is mostly true. Then he would say, "All we have to do is measure your genotype and we will know all about you." I would say, "Untrue." Because when you start with DNA, the DNA makes RNA and the messenger RNA must move from the gene through the nuclear pores to the cytoplasm where it will be converted into proteins.

> **Now, as a DNA genotyper is looking at your genes, he is only going to know that you start off with a collection of genes. He is not going to know if those genes successfully navigate the cellular environment to become a product.**

It would be like going to an automobile manufacturer and saying, "I see you have dozens of designs for next year's Chevy Camaro, so we now know exactly what you will be selling next year." The designers might say, "No you don't. We are not sure which of these designs will actually go into production."

The genotypers are out there examining a model that never went into production because in the end, the cell did not choose to make it. It did not convert that particular gene into a product. So the genotype guys are picking up the earliest levels of information, before anyone has weighed in and decided whether it is ever going to go anywhere.

That is just one problem. Another problem that I think is even more pressing is that many cancers are not driven by mutations at all. That is the ultimate fallacy of genotypic analyses—that cancers use only mutated genes. Cancers probably, more often, use normal genes in abnormal ways.

So many cancers may actually over-express or mis-regulate normal genes. If that is the case, how in the world are you going to prove that cancer is a cancer, if it is just using the normal PI3K or the normal MEK/ERK pathway in an abnormal way??

Q: Is there medical literature that corroborates your opinion that functional profiling may be superior to genomic profiling?

A: Yes, but it is difficult in this environment to get papers published. I have written many interesting papers that were rejected over and over. We recently wrote a paper about lung cancer in which we doubled the response rate (30 to 64.5 percent) and nearly doubled the survival (13.5 to 21.3 months) in previously untreated Stage 4 lung cancer. You would think that would have warranted a review. This was an Institutional Review Board (IRB) approved, clinical protocol conducted at a university medical center, analyzed by the senior biostatistician at the University of California, Irvine.

After its submission to the *Journal of Thoracic Oncology*, we received it back the next day! They did not want to even consider it. I jokingly commented to my staff that I thought it might be interesting to dust the pages for fingerprints, as I was sure that no one even opened the manuscript. It was never examined, because it reported something that they did not want to hear. It seemed that they did not want the information to get out.

Do we have corroborative evidence? Absolutely, yes!

We have two very compelling meta-analyses that I helped co-author. One was published in *Blood*, the American Society of Hematology's journal in 2007. This meta-analysis included almost 2,000 patients with different blood-borne tumors. There was an unequivocal, statistically significant improvement in response and survival, across the board, for patients who received assay "sensitive drugs."

More recently a study published by American Society of Clinical Oncology (ASCO) in 2013 examined 2,581 prospective and retrospective analyses in a variety of solid tumors and analyzed the outcome of patients who received "active drugs" (good drugs in the test tube) versus those who received inactive drugs. The receiver operator curve achieved 0.89, the sensitivity was .92, and the specificity was .72. Patients who were given active drugs had a 2.04-fold higher response rate ($p < 0.001$) and a 1.4-fold higher one-year survival ($p < 0.02$).

There are virtually no clinical trials that have achieved that significance, yet it wasn't even accepted for a poster.

Q: How many people are doing the kind of work that you are doing—functional profiling—in the United States?

A: You can imagine that people are hesitant to take a swim in "shark infested waters." Very few investigators have departed from the molecular biology platforms to examine functional platforms. However, there are a few intrepid investigators who do so.

Years ago, my colleague Larry Weisenthal, M.D. and I started a company to do this very work, but our work was usurped by a cell-growth-based program, so I left. Dr. Weisenthal and I continue to do related work using this tissue culture platform.

There are new entrants into the field. There are a couple on the East Coast that have tried to make a go of it, but they have not had an easy time, partly because they were so convinced that if they marketed it properly, the scientists would come around. They dedicated enormous resources to selling this platform, but people were still looking askance, even at reasonable data. They were not coming around.

There are a small coterie of investigators around the world, groups in Amsterdam, England, Northern Europe, Germany, Japan and us, who are continuing to do the work, because it is effective.

Once you see results from our laboratory model, which regularly doubles the survival and outcomes of generic clinical oncology, it is very difficult to go back and use the textbook.

We are twice as good as anyone else. This is a very defensible statement, measured by response and survival rates.

Q: How often do your results differ from genomic profiling tests?

A: We are here to save lives. This is not a zero sum game. What we want for patients is information. If a gene profile identifies a particular marker that looks like it might be of use, and I test the patient against a particular chemo combination to find the patient has a very appealing profile of dose response to the drugs that the genomic profile identifies, I am happy. That is a good thing.

However, just because you carry a particular mutation or amplification, does not mean that you will respond to that particular drug. However, if you are sensitive to one of those drugs, the likelihood is that you will respond. Let me give you an example. There was a paper published in the November, 2010 *Journal of Clinical Oncology* where they chose chemotherapeutic drugs for previously treated patients based on genomic profiling. The drug brought about only a 10 percent response rate. Virtually all of their responders were breast and ovarian cancer patients.

Our response rate for that same population of heavily pre-treated refractory ovarian and breast cancer patients is 50 percent, not 10

percent. Our functional platform is a much closer approximation of patient responsiveness than the simple profile of their genetic information. It is a much more robust platform.

Q: Have you treated patients who were essentially told, prior to meeting you, "Get your affairs in order," or "Call hospice," whose outcomes belied the previous prognoses? Can you give some examples?

A: Yes, all the time. For example, one of my patients in his late 40s had non-small cell lung cancer. He was treated through a major University's program in Los Angeles and received opinions from a major hospital in Los Angeles, as well. He received a very standard platinum-based chemotherapy regimen. He did well for a period of months, and then he got much worse. They put him on hospice care.

Subsequently, he heard about me and came to my office. We did a biopsy, and discovered he had a profile of relative sensitivity to a specific chemotherapy regimen. He came to me for his treatments as he was in hospice care and they were not supposed to treat him. He would drive down from West Los Angeles and was fine for a year.

After one year, he developed pain in his abdomen. I re-staged him and realized he had a large mass in his abdomen, a metastatic recurrence. The lung was under control. At that point, most people would say, "I guess that hospice care was correct for you." I said, "No, no, no, let's take this out and figure out what to do." So we biopsied him again, this time he had an unexpected profile for Tarceva. I gave him Tarceva and now, 11 years since diagnosis, he is doing well.

He told me, "I am the longest living metastatic non-small cell lung cancer patient in the history of the Veterans Administration."

Q: Is it fair to say that most of the chemotherapy drugs you prescribe are "off label," not what is typically used?

A: That is not necessarily true. For example, the most recent lung cancer paper that we published had patients with newly diagnosed non-small cell lung cancer. They received compendium-listed, FDA-approved, insurance-authorized chemotherapy. There was not a single new drug in the mix, yet the response rate was double and the survival rate was nearly double, just by reconfiguring the existing FDA-approved compendium-listed drugs.

Q: Do you ever run into insurance companies that won't cover your protocol?

A: We run into it more and more. That is a policy issue. I can't change the reimbursement environment; I can only find the right thing to do. Some patients pay out of their pocket, some patients unfortunately can't get the drugs.

I worked with a patient from Alberta, Canada who came to me with recurrent ovarian cancer. The drugs worked perfectly. The health care system would not pay for it in Alberta. Her case was so compelling that the province of Alberta, seeing that it worked so well, changed their reimbursement policy to include our combination.

Q: Regarding people who get tested by your laboratory, how does the process work to begin the "testing process"?

A: Every cancer patient is diagnosed based upon tissue.

No one is treated based upon x-rays or blood tests, unless it is leukemia. The point is, this is an opportunity to figure out not only what the patient has, but what to do about it.

There is virtually no single treatment for any disease. In most settings, cancers are managed with many different options. You must tell the surgeon to send sterile excess tissue samples to our laboratory by overnight courier. Seven days later we have results. Some people say they don't want to wait, but the fact is when you visit your doctor, you need to wait anyway. Your doctor is not treating you that week. Frequently they need to put in a port-o-cath, do a biopsy, complete staging, do an MRI, evaluate tumor markers, do your biochemical workup, and engage in all kinds of things between the time that you are diagnosed and the time you actually get treated.

Q: How many chemotherapy drugs and chemotherapy drug combinations do you test?

A: The standard profile is 16 drugs and combinations.

> **However, there are some absolutes. We know some combinations don't work in certain cancers. There are some general guidelines.**

We try to provide the doctors with information consistent with what they are interested in using. We touch on those combinations. We try to conform to the general experience of each given disease. The 16 drugs and combinations usually cover the bases.

Q: Dr. Ralph Moss commented in his book, *Customized Cancer Treatment*, about laboratories in Europe that are testing blood versus tissue samples. Any thoughts on this matter?

A: These are gene tests. They are isolating Circulating Tumor Cells (CTC) and they are doing genomics. They are looking to see if the CTCs have a particular target gene.

This is a blood test, picking targets based on genes. Even given the luxury of ample tissue samples from a surgical biopsy, the folks at a major cancer research institute in the Southwest, using similar genomic analyses, only came up with a 10 percent response rate. I hardly expect gene profiles, based upon isolated CTCs, will produce a better response rate than that.

Q: What is your attitude about other treatments or therapies that some integrative doctors and practitioners recommend such as: nutritional recommendations, evidence-based supplementation regarding specific botanicals, vitamins or extracts, exercise regimens, mind-body approaches, and other therapies that may help bring about better outcomes?

A: First, I would say, anything that works for patients should be explored.

From the standpoint of non-chemotherapeutic treatments, non-allopathic therapy, there is a wealth of scientific data to support the concept of lifestyle change, dietary impact, and other interventions to assist patients as they confront cancer.

Many of the practitioners may provide these treatments in a way that, on some occasions, discourages patients from seeking other types of treatments. I am a little hesitant to have patients eschew what may be active in favor of natural therapies, because many natural therapies are not curative.

Most of the natural therapies have active ingredients and are based on sound science. We know that a number of different compounds can induce immunological responses. They can have effects on metabolism. We know that curcuminoids and other agents are very interesting, with many interesting biological properties. But, many of these compounds are not highly potent and it can be difficult to get bioavailability. For example, curcuminoids are generally not well absorbed, even though they are active. Many of these other therapies can, however, help people feel better.

Many cancer centers of the world are now rushing into the complementary care field, as if they invented complementary care. These are exactly the things that practitioners in this field have been espousing for decades. There is no question, there is something to complementary care, and there is no question that people benefit from it. It should be combined with other things. I don't think it should be an "either/or" proposition.

Q: Do you think the implementation of integrative therapies at the cancer centers may be related to branding and marketing?

A: Yes, I do.

Q: Will you collaborate or work with other doctors or scientists who have expertise in other complementary treatment methodologies that may help strengthen the patients' immune system?

A: Yes. For example, I have worked with Dr. Keith Block for many years. Also, I was very impressed with the level of sophistication of the medical integrative oncologists I met at the medical symposium I attended (Healthy Medicine Academy) in Scottsdale last year. Many of them are more scientifically sophisticated with regard to cellular biology and metabolomics than many of the academic oncologists. The level of sophistication was quite impressive.

Q: Where do you see cancer research and clinical treatments going in the future? Specifically, is there any current research in the laboratories or in clinical practices that show great promise to eradicate, control, or seriously mitigate cancer's continuing threat to human life?

A: I think the investment in genomics, and the abandonment of biochemistry, has led to 50 years of a collection of scientists who were experts at doing DNA analysis, but have lost any understanding of biochemical principles.

Cancer is not information; it is a phenomenon. Many of these scientists don't understand science. They are pattern recognition people. There are very few biochemists.

Q: Any parting words or pearls of wisdom that you'd like to impart to people currently diagnosed with cancer or who are not responding to current treatments and therapies?

A: Every cancer patient is unique.

> **There is no textbook guideline or principle that will tell how a given patient will respond. Statistics apply to populations, not individuals.**

When a patient is diagnosed, their doctor can only fall back on population statistics. Patients must realize they are "round pegs" being banged into the square holes of the doctor's guidelines. If they are lucky, they squeeze through the hole, and if they are not they get a lot of hits on the head with chemotherapy that does not work, while their doctor is trying to prove that they belong in the wrong hole. Patients must say to their doctor:

> **"I am going to have only one chance to get first-line chemotherapy and I know that first-line chemotherapy is my best chance of being cured. Show me evidence that I am likely to do better than the average person, I want something that makes me 'un-average.'"**

That is a tissue culture platform that will identify the likelihood of response and improve their outcome twofold. Period. Statistically, significantly improve their outcome. For recurring patients, the doctors are admittedly unaware of what to do. If your doctor doesn't know what to do, you really have to worry about what will happen. They will put you on anything you have not had. It is a crapshoot.

> **So from our standpoint, whether it is newly diagnosed patients or recurring patients, an appropriately conducted laboratory study of our type, or related, will double the response rate.**

If it is someone who has a 30 to 40 percent chance starting off, we will push him or her up to 60, 70, or 80 percent. If it is someone who has recurrent cancer, and a dismal prognosis, say a 10 or 20 percent chance, we will push them up to a 30, 40 or 50 percent chance.

Also, we will provide any patient who runs up against resistance with their doctor, documentation of the predictive validity of our tests. If their doctor can prove that what we are doing is not working, I want to talk to them. It is always better with our tests, but it is not perfect.

Q: Any final thoughts?

A: This is a very exciting time in oncology and we want to give each patient his or her best chance to get better.

DONALD YANCE, JR., C.N., M.H.

ABOUT DONALD YANCE, JR., C.N., M.H. An internationally recognized expert in botanical and nutritional medicine, Donald Yance, Jr., C.N., M.H., has devoted his life to developing a unique approach to health and healing. Known as Donnie, he works primarily with cancer issues and combines his passion for the latest scientific research with the wisdom of healing traditions. He is a certified nutritionist and clinical master herbalist.

Yance is the founder of the Mederi Foundation which is dedicated to the transformation of healthcare. The Mederi Centre for Natural Healing is a clinic he founded where a "whole systems" approach combines botanical and nutritional medicines as primary therapies best suited for the individual. Yance is also the formulator and president of Natura Health Products, a line of advanced botanical and nutritional products.

This healer wrote two books: *Herbal Medicine, Healing and Cancer* (Keats Publishing, 1999), and, *Adaptogens in Medical Herbalism: Elite Herbs and Natural Compounds for Mastering Stress, Aging, and Chronic Disease* (Healing Arts Press, 2013).

Throughout more than 25 years of clinical practice, Yance's philosophy and practice have evolved into the integrative model that he calls the Eclectic Triphasic Medical System (ETMS). This system is a distinctive approach to healing that calls for the integration of traditional, wholistic medicine with modern, allopathic medicine—thus creating a custom-tailored approach for each individual that relies on scientific research, logic, common sense, and intuitive wisdom. The primary goal of ETMS, according to Yance, is to bring the body into harmonious balance with nontoxic or low-toxicity, target-specific, disease-suppressing agents. This is achieved through the application of synergistic herbal and nutritional formulations (naturally phytochemically complex medicines), dietary therapeutics, and other specific therapies as indicated.

Interview

Q: What motivated you to devote your career to enhancing healing and wellness, especially regarding cancer patients?

A: It started in high school. A cousin sent me a book entitled *Back to Eden*. It is an old book about herbal medicine, the folkloric usage of herbs. The book struck a chord in my heart. The concept that plants were left here by our Creator to provide remedies to support our health resonated with me.

As a junior in high school, I worked in a natural food store. Later on, in 1987, I became part owner of another natural food store and ran its supplement section. In the course of accumulating knowledge, I opened a clinic offering recommendations to patients and consumers seeking advice about herbal and nutritional approaches to health issues. I obtained a degree in nutritional medicine, continually studied herbs, started going to naturopathic conferences between 1987 and 1993, and attended the first American Herbalist Guild Symposium in 1989.

I learned over time that I had an ability to "touch" the hearts of people with cancer and became devoted to helping cancer patients get well.

In the late 1980s, I worked with a patient named Sinclair. She had a mastectomy, chemotherapy, and was young, in her 30s. She had Stage 4 breast cancer. I did everything I could to keep her alive, but ultimately, she died. Her family gave me a ring that she made for me. I still wear it on my hand to this day. She helped me examine myself, to look inside, and invigorated my desire to devote myself to the pursuit of healing.

Q: What does the concept "ETMS" stand for? What are the core tenets that form the foundation of ETMS, and how does this concept work?

A: ETMS stands for Eclectic Triphasic Medical System. We also call it "Mederi Medicine." Mederi means "to heal and become whole" in Latin and is the name of my foundation which includes my clinical practice where I apply the ETMS. It is a blueprint of my approach; it is a comprehensive, holistic model that stems from my underlying philosophy of how we help people deal with cancer. Much of my work, my decisions and perspectives, comes from my personal experience in actual clinical practice as well as my scientific research.

We implement a plan or protocol using what I call the five ETMS 'toolboxes.' These include botanical, nutritional, dietary, lifestyle, and to the extent possible, ETMS-guided pharmaceutical medicines (as opposed to the 'standard of care').

As we develop the protocol, we are thinking strategically about the short-term, intermediate and long- term objectives. Because modern conventional medicine is based solely on rational thought, it is intellectual, scholastic, standardized, predictable, and sometimes emotional in character (fear-driven, whereby doctors worry about the legal consequences of not following the "standard of care" and patients worry about everything from the cancer itself to the treatments proposed by the oncologist). The result is often less than therapeutic for the body, mind, and soul.

In contrast, the ETMS merges ancient wisdom, modern research, and introspective prayer. I think of this process as the cross-pollination of rational-intellectual reasoning with meditative prayer, blending all that we know with what is still unknown in the realm of healing.

Regarding the word 'Eclectic', in holistic medicine, instead of focusing on a single root cause and attempting to find a magic bullet solution, it is essential to address all of the root causes.

The term 'eclectic' means that we consider a variety of therapeutic options, always in the best interest of getting the patient well. One type of treatment therapy is too reductionist for a disease as complex as cancer.

In the field of holistic medicine, we have many useful therapies to employ, but knowing which ones and how to combine them, and especially to integrate them with conventional medicine, takes expertise and skill. Regarding 'Triphasic':

We are talking about three branches, which include the host, the microenvironment, and the cancer itself.

The host (patient) and what we do about the person is most critical. We engage in a comprehensive host assessment. A great portion of the medicine is used to create the highest state of health in that person whether they have disease or not. We engage in critical thinking, actively and skillfully conceptualizing, analyzing and synthesizing information that we gather from observation, learning about symptoms and the patient's history.

We assess the microenvironment, using various bio-marker laboratory tests, most of which are blood tests.

We don't do any tests unless they are relevant to the situation and are substantiated by solid scientific data. We analyze test results to help inform us of something we need to do therapeutically. We don't do fringe tests. For example, testing can be useful to assess vitamin D levels (both 25 OH and 125 diOPH forms) in the blood, angiogenic activity as well as hyper-thrombosis. We look at multiple areas and "shift problematic issues" to promote the health of the host. We alter these areas so they cannot be "hijacked" by the tumor. A cancer cell cannot do any harm, nor grow into a tumor, unless it is taking control of the microenvironment.

We want to change all of the markers we discover to be the most conducive to the host and the least conducive to the tumor or the cancer. There is a constant tug of war over the microenvironment. If the cancer is winning that tug of war, the patient is in big trouble. We continually work to shift that as much as possible. This is the second branch of the triphasic approach.

The third branch is the cancer itself.

Now we are looking at the phenotype of the tumor, not necessarily the genotype. Genotyping, also called gene sequencing, is very trendy now and people don't know how to interpret that information. We are looking at protein expression, micro-gene analysis.

There are many different ways we look at the phenotype of the cancer. All cancers are alike, but they are alike in unique ways. For example, one person may have breast cancer that is ER/PR positive and she may do absolutely nothing therapeutically, be diagnosed at 65 years old, and live another 25 years to 90, ultimately dying from a non-cancer cause. A different woman may be diagnosed with the same breast cancer, be treated aggressively with standard of care medicine, and be dead within one or two years.

They both were staged the same, classified the same, were the same age, but can have vastly different outcomes.

This can happen for many reasons. There are a lot of characteristics within the phenotype that describe what I refer to as the "intelligence of the cancer." Phenotype is like the personality of the cancer, the cancer traits that lead to its proliferative, angiogenic status and what makes it intelligent.

Cancer needs a cooperative environment to manifest. That's not to say that it cannot manipulate even a healthy environment, because it can; it is just more likely if the terrain is more favorable or more conducive to its ability to thrive.

If a person's cancer phenotype is highly proliferative and intelligent in nature, and that person has a very poor internal environment, the cancer will most likely spread quickly. In contrast, if the person has a healthy internal environment, he or she will be better equipped to fight even a very smart cancer. That same person with poor health can also manifest cancer of a less aggressive phenotype or character, and live many years despite it.

So, once we've assessed the three branches—the host, the microenvironment, and the cancer—we consider the patient's treatment options. I want to know if a therapy will be helpful; I want to know what the upside will be if we do chemo or radiation. Present cancer treatment strategies are based on the assumption that a therapy may work ("response") or not work ("no response"). However, the existing evidence suggests that current cancer treatment modalities may also have a cancer-promoting effect in some patients.

In some cases surgery, radiation, chemotherapy and immunotherapy can stimulate tumor growth/metastatic spread and decrease survival.

When cancer cells are resistant to chemotherapy or radiation, these treatments are doing harm. I believe that results of cancer treatment may be improved by detection and use, with careful interpretation, of an array of biomarkers that correlate with positive or negative therapeutic effects.

There are ways to look at tumor biomarkers based on molecular profiling coupled with chemosensitivity resistance tests from the Weisenthal Cancer Group or Rational Therapeutics; both are located in Southern California. I don't use either of them by themselves. I overlap the data.

I also look at blood and genetic abnormalities that can be somewhat predictive of the sensitivity of the drug and toxicity. Now we can know if the drug is highly toxic, because a person's liver does not break it down well. We can also know if the tumor is highly sensitive to the drug.

The solution is, you take the drug at half the dosage of standard of care; it is still a lot of drug, but you don't need to deal with the excessive toxicity of the drug.

Q: When people think of botanical-therapeutic approaches, some are quite skeptical as to whether "plants, plant extracts and combinations of plant medicine" can have a profound, compelling impact on cancer. How would you address such skepticism?

A: There is no herbal cure for cancer. Many people postulate that herbs cure cancer without understanding the specifics of the person's situation. You can't just take an herb and think that you will be cured. You must apply a model that is based in herbal medicine. You must have a relationship with your patient and the medicines you use as well.

Anyone who promises a 'cure' through adopting a radical diet or this week's miracle remedy (currently, it's cannabis) is making false promises. However, and this is important, the allopathic doctor who discourages patients from any therapies other than conventional chemotherapy and radiation is just as unhelpful as the radical alternative practitioner or institution that promotes IV vitamin C and hydrogen peroxide infusions or wheat grass implants.

I believe both of those stances are radically shortsighted, and definitely not in the best interest of the patient. For example, the first thing an allopathic doctor (and often, the patient) wants is to remove the cancer by cutting it out. They don't recognize that cancer is systemic, and often spreads as a result of aggressive localized treatments.

Modern conventional medicine tries and wants desperately to understand and quantify the concept of "curing disease," which is in stark contrast to the healing philosophy of the ETMS and traditional medicine. For example, we are brainwashed into believing that the quick eradication of a tumor is curative, when what actually cures people is providing patients with a significantly longer and higher quality of life beyond what they otherwise would experience. Tumor eradication does not equal a significantly longer and higher quality of life, but the promise of eradication impresses people.

A new drug can make the headlines of every newspaper, because it offers new hope for curing cancer. The term "breakthrough" is often used in these headlines; frequently it is erroneously used.

The truth? Even the best drugs are only extending the lives of people two to three months. These drugs often cause significant side effects and diminish quality of life, while costing many thousands of dollars per month.

**The scientific data is overwhelming on the benefits
of herbs in oncology. Overwhelming.**

Herbs work in a very complex manner. We know certain compounds in single herbs can affect hundreds of signal pathways involving cancer. They work to down-regulate certain genes. They work at the mutational level, they work at the intercellular level, they work at the cell receptor level; they also work at the extra-cellular level.

The same herb can protect healthy cells, vital organs and tissues from chemo, and it can also potentiate the chemo so it works better against the cancer cells, as well as inhibit multi-drug resistance. It also inhibits the ability of the cancer cell to build resistance to the chemotherapy.

Herbs can also do the following: down-regulate certain growth factors, change the fibrolynic pathways, bolster natural killer cells, support the innate immune system, activate dendritic cells, affect thrombosis, impact hormones, down-regulate drug resistance pumps, bring about oxidative damage to cancer cells, target all kinds of resistance mechanisms concerning chemo and protect healthy cells.

There are all kinds of data, real credible data, supporting these actions. No oncologist can refute these assertions.

**Herbs are foundational to the healing protocol that I recom-
mend for everyone. As a traditional herbalist, I believe that
'the sum of all the parts is greater than any single part.'**

For this reason, I prescribe combinations of herbs and herbal isolates customized to the individual. This includes using whole herbs, herbal extracts, super concentrated herbal extracts, and herbal isolates. I use herbs internally as teas, tincture formulas, and concentrated extracts in liquids and capsules.

I always combine a powdered extract, either a 4:1 or 8:1 concentration with an isolate. I do this for several reasons: First, the beneficial effects are often superior and more diverse than the single isolate; second, the plant often contains compounds that buffer or reduce the harshness or potential toxicity that the isolate may possess; and third, out of respect for the gift of the whole herb.

I believe herbs offer the most of any of the tools in the toolbox to accomplish longevity and quality of life.

Q: It concerns me when a doctor makes the sweeping statement: "You are cured," or "You are cancer free." I believe it can be misleading to a patient and give them a false sense of security. Thoughts?

A: We all have cancer stem cells. There is no way to know where they are located based upon the diagnostic tools we have today. Quite often, the cancer can come back even more aggressively, or as a different cancer phenotype after allopathic treatments such as chemotherapy and radiation therapy. A lot of collateral damage can be done with the allopathic toolbox. Treatments must be highly targeted to the patient's cancer.

Contrary to many doctors' opinions, I don't think surgery is the best initial, upfront therapy. It can only be a cure for cancers that are indolent in nature and that don't express metastatic characteristics. Otherwise, it can provoke systemic tumor growth and weaken the host. However, I am not saying we should not do surgery, as a general statement. It is all about the timing and what else you are doing.

We need to plan carefully 'when' surgery should happen and prep the person systemically by strengthening them with anabolic-immune-enhancing botanicals and immuno-nutrients for an appropriate period of time before, as well as after, the surgery.

It is critical that we learn what kind of cancer the individual has, put together a protocol that strengthens the host, strengthens the terrain that targets the tumor, and see what effect it has systemically. After providing systemic therapy, surgery can now be less invasive due to a systemic protocol that can dramatically shrink the tumor, prior to surgery. We effectively alter a systemic disease, systemically, first and foremost. This approach is in the long-term best interest of the patient as far as reducing the chance of a recurrence.

Q: Based on your comments, I assume you prefer a metronomic approach to chemotherapy, whereby the distribution of the chemo drug(s) is at a lower dose?

A: Ideally, we want pharmaceutical (allopathic) medicine to cause the most damage to the cancer and the least damage to the host.

If it is not the right kind of allopathic medicine, or the dose is too high, the toxicity ultimately causes excessive damage to the healthy cells, sometimes in spite of all we do to protect the host. In most cases, the patient embarks upon a strict standard of care chemotherapy, frequently at a higher dose than they may be able to tolerate, and does not obtain the best tests to determine what may be the best chemotherapy or other treatments for the particular cancer. So, frequently, the treatment only works for a smaller quantity of people, at random, and the majority may encounter immense suffering with little or no reduction of their tumor.

It is a philosophical strategy. With a fast growing, proliferative cancer, a young person may be able to handle more toxicity; therefore, it may make sense to use dosages a little larger than metronomic. However, with most people past the age of 50, with intermediate growing tumors, it makes more sense to think metronomically and to think in a synergistic manner.

Not only do I think in terms of biological agents and chemotherapy, but I also may advise patients to ask their oncologist about "out of the box" drugs like: Rapamiacin (an mTOR inhibitor), Metformin (an insulin sensitizer that activates AMPK), Celebrex (a COX -2 inhibitor used primarily for arthritis), Tagamet (a histamine type-2 receptor antagonist), Tetrathiomolybdate (a copper-chelating drug with anti-antiogenic effects) and Chloroquine (a CXCR4 inhibitor).

My preference is always lower doses of chemotherapeutic drugs in combination with herbs which bring about incredible synergistic results.

Q: Are there certain types of natural agents, vitamins, extracts or combinations of natural agents that are prevalent and most useful in fighting cancer, or, does each type of cancer and/or person require a different approach?

A: I usually start by building a foundation with herbs that are normalizing, non-specific, and overall protective. The underlying theme of herbs in this category is to build up the host so he or she can facilitate energy more efficiently and create a reservoir of energy. By improving the ability of the body to eliminate toxins, we bring about an anti-toxic effect.

We work with adaptogenic remedies, as well as other remedies. Adaptogenic formulations include primary adaptogens and adaptogen companion extracts such as: rosemary, ginger, green tea, turmeric, and sage, many of which are culinary herbs. They won't have an immediate, profound effect, but we will "bathe" the body, the cells, with lots of phytonutrition that is made up of many phenolic compounds which I couple with primary adaptogens and, sometimes, a few protective things from the sulfur family like broccoli sprouts, cabbage sprouts, or wasabi. These contain other unique compounds that everyone will derive benefits from.

Also, we recommend companion nutrients that aid in the adaptogenic effect like anabolic botanicals. Some are food concentrates like a non-denatured (unpasteurized) whey protein powder that is from free-range grass fed cattle. This provides an array of efficiently utilized, high quality protein. Other things like colostrum, chlorella and barley grass bring massive amounts of nutrients to the body that offer general non-specific support.

Once the foundation is in place for prevention and general care, the dosage is adjusted. Healthy people only take small amounts of these things. Chronically ill people take more. Seriously ill people take an abundance (especially plant medicine) at much higher doses and concentrations. At least three to four times per day, the patient needs to take certain specific agents to bring about a sufficient shift, especially with ill people, to turn the corner.

Q: I have heard some people say that herbs are only supportive and not cytotoxic. Regarding prevalent agents, are some supportive in nature while others are cytotoxic, meaning they kill cancer cells?

A: Herbs are pleotrophic, meaning they are multi-taskers, and are often doing a multitude of things to benefit us. Some are supportive (to the host), while others are cytotoxic. Some are both.

> **Some herbs of course are more supportive and tonic-like, normalizing cell behavior, while cytotoxic ones are well, shall we say 'offensive minded' and capable of selectively inducing apoptosis (cell death) to abnormal cancer cells, both directly as well as indirectly.**

Many chemotherapeutic drugs are derived from plants like the Pacific yew tree (*Taxus brevifolia*), Madagasgar periwinkle (*Catharanthus roseus*), and May apple tree (*Podophyllum peltatum*), and others.

I use all of these as whole-plant extracts as well, which can both potentiate the chemotherapy and reduce drug resistance, because of the many added complementary compounds in the whole plant. A plant is a complex entity, and usually has as many as 100 active compounds working synergistically and effectively against cancer cells.

We need to think in harmony; that nourishing the body is critical. We need to work backwards from the standard medical model, which attacks the symptoms and the cancer.

The standard perspective is "we need to get the cancer out of our body, or we need to radiate it." We need to think philosophically, differently. We need to nourish and balance the body to make the cancer go into remission or go away. If we cannot make peace with the body, then we may need to implement a joint strategy of becoming more "offensive" with cancer with the natural toolbox and the allopathic (standard) toolbox together.

In a younger person, cancer is created, generally, from genomic abnormalities and less from a lifetime of poor lifestyle habits that you find in an older person.

I want to know more about the proliferative and aggressive nature of the cancer. I want to know more about "the intelligence of the cancer." We look at proliferative cancer markers. The Ki67 antigen tumor marker test is one example.

With younger people, as I mentioned earlier, sometimes it makes sense to be more offensive with a robust protocol, including cytotoxic agents, which may include allopathic tools. Neoadjunctive therapy (therapy given before the main treatment to shrink the size of the tumor) is an important strategy to consider. Again, as I stated earlier, it is very important that systemic therapy be done prior to surgery and radiation.

Slowly, today, more chemo is being done neoadjunctively, before surgery and the excision of cancer. It is a slow moving philosophy. The concept that you must get the cancer out immediately before it spreads does not make sense.

There is no rush. It is better to get the data you need first, unless the cancer is discovered at such a late stage, whereby the tumor may be impeding an area that brings about a life-threatening situation. Short of that, it is better to do systemic work first.

Q: How personalized or customized are your recommendations when you develop a comprehensive treatment plan?

A: Our recommendations are very personalized. Approximately 50 percent of our recommendations are personalized with the goal of supporting and improving the health of the host. Multiple tests give me extra information. I build the host, constitutionally. Approximately 50 percent of our recommendations are standardized.

Let me give you an example: Four years ago a woman in her 40s had HER2/neu positive breast cancer and ovarian cancer. Tumors continued to grow aggressively despite her chemotherapy treatment. I did a molecular workup on her tumor. She was also tested through the Weisenthal Cancer Group.

I advised that she should not engage in any more chemo, but I suggested that she consider an oral medication, Tykerb, then a newer drug for breast cancer. The standard dosage is five pills per day. I advised her to ask her oncologist about a lower dose of three per day, with a 10 days on and four days off regimen. All other therapeutic interventions were botanical. She had no toxicity and all the tumors disappeared. She was then able to reduce her pills from three to two per day. I monitored her for two years.

Then, a year and a half ago, she suddenly stopped communicating. I had no more contact with her. Just recently, she came in and was not feeling well. Her neurological symptoms were significant. She had a scan indicating tumors all over her brain and her liver was bulging out. She had stopped all of the drugs and botanicals, several months prior. She said, "I felt fine and thought I was fine." She continued, "The oncologist wants me to do radiation on my brain, resect my liver and wants me on several drugs." I said, "Wait, wait, wait! We had something that was working very well." I looked at her blood regarding her serum HER2/neu level. No doctor looks at blood for HER2/neu, but there is so much scientific literature, at least 12 studies, showing validity regarding whether a HER2/neu patient will respond to a particular drug. In my practice, obtaining this information and knowing what to do with it has resulted in saving the lives of five or six women who were in the same situation. I have found that this test is the most accurate way to determine if the HER2/neu is a good up-regulated receptor and a good target to go after. This test is not done in any cancer center in the country, yet.

So, in this woman's case, I suggested she go back on Tykerb to target her HER2/neu, combined with a more aggressive botanical regimen, and one other drug. After just five weeks, her neurological symptoms disappeared and her liver was clear of tumors. This one blood test showed a target that enabled us to individualize both the holistic and conventional therapies effectively.

We do these kinds of things all the time. For some it is quite an involved process. If people are compliant, I believe we can bring about great outcomes with the great majority of people, regardless of their prognosis.

> **Q: Are there certain tests, i.e., blood tests you use and other diagnostic tests, not generally accepted by conventional medicine, that your experience shows can be determinative of the existence of cancer, the progression of cancer, and that lead you to make specific recommendations?**

A: There are lots of valuable laboratory tests. There are a host of tumor biomarkers helpful to assess if a treatment is working, if the cancer is progressing or if someone has cancer. There are markers indicative of specific growth factors that relate to the cancer, bone marrow health and other critical factors. However, tests are useless unless you know how to interpret them. This is a real problem.

Several recent scientific studies have come out demonstrating that people with low levels of vitamin D, upon discovering they have cancer, have significantly worse outcomes versus those who had higher vitamin D levels. This includes colorectal, breast, prostate and lymphomas, and probably correlates with other cancers, as well. Researchers have also found that higher levels of circulating vitamin D on diagnosis of cancer are associated with significantly better survival and remission rates.

The preferable range for cancer patients regarding the vitamin D level is between 50 to 80 ng/ml. This can be determined by having a 25 (OH) Hydroxy Vitamin D test. Additionally, one should also look at the 1,25 Dihydroxy Vitamin D test or you can overdose on vitamin D. The results of the 25 and 125 test should be approximately the same number: in the 50 to 80 range. You don't want to hyper-calcify. To minimize the possibility of hyper-calcifying you should eat natto (fermented soybeans) a Japanese food, for its vitamin K. Also, the vitamin K2 can be helpful for bone health and the liver.

Evidence from observational studies indicates inverse associations of circulating 25 (OH) Hydroxy Vitamin D with risks of death due to cardiovascular disease, cancer, and other causes. Supplementation with vitamin D3 significantly reduces overall mortality among older adults.

Another recent study, reported by researchers at the 36th Annual San Antonio Breast Cancer Symposium, found that patients with HER2/neu positive breast cancer who receive vitamin D supplementation during the course of their treatment appear to have significantly better outcomes than patients who don't take the supplements.

Many people and most cancer patients are deficient in zinc, vitamin D, and selenium. There are tests to assess these issues, so deficiencies can be addressed. Also, fibrolynic and angiogenesis issues can be assessed with specific tests, providing us with useful information.

There is a massive amount of medical literature supporting the importance of these tests and many other tests we use to gather valuable information.

Q: Many mainstream doctors and scientists will not acknowledge any types of treatment as potentially acceptable unless they pass the placebo-controlled, randomized, double-blind, large, Phase 3, FDA study procedures. What constitutes real science or evidence, or "enough evidence," supporting the recommendation of specific alternative treatments?

A: The conventional medical system has poor evidence regarding treatments that conventional practitioners administer. What is the evidence, I ask, regarding aggressive up-front surgeries or radiation therapy when they fry the cervix? Numerous studies confirm that radiation therapy increases the risk of second malignancies.

I do believe all of these conventional treatments including radiation therapy have a place in cancer

**therapy, but they need to be used more wisely under the
umbrella of a whole systems approach, such as ETMS,
that is integrative and personalized, whereby systemic
therapies are the primary focus and localized
treatments are adjunctive.**

You would be very surprised to see what little evidence there is, even with some of the so-called breakthrough biological agents that cost a fortune. For example, take the anti-prostate cancer drug Provenge (sipuleucel-T). If you have seen the television ads for Provenge, you might think it was the greatest breakthrough in prostate cancer treatment. It's not, and it might not even be as good as the results demonstrated in the clinical trials that got it approved.

In April of 2010, the FDA approved Provenge for advanced prostate cancer, satisfying investors in Dendreon (the manufacturer) and patients who for years had demanded the drug be put on the market. The conclusions derived from the study were very weak, at best. Earlier studies did not prove that Provenge extended people's lives. One study showing slight improvement was pushed through the FDA. It brought about a two-month extension in survival versus previous studies.

**Generally, the medical studies and associated medical
literature cited to support conventional medical therapies, including chemotherapy, for pancreatic cancer, glioblastomas, and other difficult cancers, are not anything
wonderful to 'write home about.'**

I do agree, however, we need to see good clinical data from studies coming from big universities. My case studies are not considered evidence in today's conventional world of oncology. We must find people willing to support and finance these studies. The problem is, who will reap financial benefit from these studies? Drug companies have shareholders. Who will spend huge amounts of money for a trial regarding an ETMS approach, even if it shows great benefit?

I want to demonstrate that a good integrative model can be a great break-through, more effective, with greater quality of life, providing much greater longevity. In my first book, *Herbal Medicine Healing and Cancer*, written in 1999, I was recommending aromatase inhibitors instead of Tamoxifen. The allopathic medical profession was very upset with my recommendations; however, standard of care now demonstrates that aromatase inhibitors are superior to Tamoxifen. They have less toxicity and work better.

Q: Can botanicals help mitigate the side effects of chemo and radiation without negating or compromising the intended effect of the treatments, and is there medical literature supporting this proposition?

A: There is a massive, overwhelming amount of medical literature with excellent data, both human and animal models, attesting to the proposition that botanical medicine with chemotherapy can in fact: be protective to healthy cells and organs, minimize side effects, improve recovery, potentiate the drug against the cancer cells, and inhibit drug resistance to the cancer cells. There is virtually no evidence showing interference of nutrient redox/antioxidants with chemotherapy and radiation, just some theoretical misconceptions. There is no real truth to it.

For example, during the past four years and right now, Yale University is looking at a combination of four Chinese herbs that protects against the toxicity of chemotherapy and poten-tiates the chemo in every model they use.

These results have been documented in major medical journals. The formula, PHY906, is made up of a mixture of four herbal extracts: *Glycyrrhiza uralensis* (Chinese licorice root), *Paeonia lactiflora*, *Scutelleria baicalensis*, and *Ziziphus jujube*. Together with Irinotecan, this herbal drug combination triggers specific changes that are not activated by each one alone, suggesting that the combination creates a unique tissue-specific response.

PHY906 is a traditional Chinese Medicine (TCM) formulation that has been used for 1,800 years to treat gastrointestinal maladies. Several preclinical animal model studies tested the ability of PHY906 to increase the therapeutic window of chemotherapy by decreasing its gastrointestinal side effects. Recently, it has been documented that PHY906 has strong protective effects regarding chemotherapy induced intestinal toxicity. Moreover, pre-clinical and early-phase clinical trials of PHY906 in combination with chemotherapy in patients with advanced hepatocellular carcinoma, pancreatic cancer and other gastrointestinal malignancies have yielded promising results.

There are only a couple of potential interactions that are as yet unclear. Black or green tea may inhibit protease inhibitors, but this interaction has nothing to do with how green tea affects hepatic detoxification pathways, but rather the fact that it contains tannins which bind up the protease inhibitor, thereby reducing absorption. If you want to take green tea extract with a protease inhibitor, it is good to wait three days until the drug has been fully absorbed. Evaluating drug-drug, nutrient-drug, or botanical-drug interactions based on the cytochrome P450 enzyme pathway for metabolism is difficult and often misleading.

Many times you will read scientific research papers where the author uses the word 'may' or 'suggest' regarding the potential impact of an herb; then everyone jumps on this—and assumes you should not take this herb with this drug, because there 'may' be an interaction.

Keep in mind that an interaction doesn't necessarily mean that the interaction is negative or harmful. Take St. John's wort (*Hypericum perforatum*) extract (SJWE), for example. Most of the interaction research on SJWE and various drugs, including the chemotherapeutic drug Irinotecan, have demonstrated that SJWE (600-900 mgs daily) can reduce blood levels between 20 to 40 percent. Although SJWE decreased blood levels of Irinotecan, it appears to increase effectiveness, and yet it decreases side effects, improves tolerability, and may even improve response rates, because of its pleotrophic anti-cancer effects.

Results of a recent study demonstrated that the SJWE significantly enhanced the tumor inhibition rate of the chemotherapeutic drug, 5-FU, improved the immune function, reduced the toxic effects and prolonged the survival time in the tumor-bearing mice. This study found a synergistic tumor-inhibiting effect of SJWE with 5-FU, and a reduction of the toxic side effects.

Oncologists often cherry-pick one obscure *in vitro* study that shows theoretically that there may be an interaction, while ignoring, or not knowing about the 29 studies that show that it works synergistically. They frequently hang their hat on that one obscure study.

The immense quantity of evidence we have, including our great depth of clinical experience spanning approximately 30 years, strongly suggests that herbs can be of great benefit for cancer patients by:

1. Helping the body cope with the side effects of chemotherapy agents.

2. Protecting bone marrow, blood, and vital organs from toxicity.

3. Enhancing immune response.

4. Potentiating the cytotoxic effects of conventional cancer treatments.

5. Inhibiting drug resistance (M.D.R/Pgp/Bcl-2/NF-kB etc.).

6. Suppressing cancer through multiple mechanisms including inner cellular gene pathways, cell surface receptors, and extra cellular signaling.

7. Supporting healing of many secondary health conditions: diabetes, CVD, insomnia, depression, pain, digestive distress, and the detrimental effects of cancer treatments on hair and skin.

8. Enhancing quality of life and lifespan.

Q: Regarding the recommendation of taking certain botanicals and extracts in a particular cancer-fighting regimen, are the concepts of dosage, bioavailability (absorption), timing, and the nature of the specific brand important?

A: Absolutely yes! The quality of the herb is critical.

In my opinion, 90 percent of the supplements on the shelf are junk. You need to know "the process" of how the herbs reach your front door from their origins. A common problem when buying herbs and nutritional agents (vitamins, minerals, amino acids, fatty acids, etc.) is differentiating between high quality, mediocre quality, and poor quality products. Too often, people buy herbal and nutritional supplements because of marketing, price, or the recommendation of a store clerk.

All of the following key factors must be considered to consistently produce high quality and effective herbal preparations:

1. Genetic factors (correct and specific species).

2. Environmental factors.

3. Climate.

4. Soil characteristics (pH, fertilization, heavy metals).

5. Infections (insects, pests, microbes); exposure activates the plant's immune system, triggering the production of various compounds (i.e., stilbene compounds like resveratrol).

6. Harvest time.

7. Parts of the plant used.

8. Duration of time from when the herb is harvested to extraction (fresh or dried).

9. Processing (pulverization, extraction, solvent polarity, temperature, duration, distillation, fermentation, purification).

10. Storage (light, oxygen, humidity, temperature).

The comparison of standardized products with reproducible chemical composition best assures reproducible pharmacologic activity. Studies show that the content of active markers in herbal products sold in health food stores can vary considerably.

Q: You own a company known as Natura Health Products that formulates botanical and nutritional products. Please tell us about this company and its purpose?

A: I have been working with cancer patients for almost 30 years. My formulations are the foundational tools in my botanical and nutritional toolboxes. I decided I wanted to bring the best botanical products possible to the marketplace. We source our products from the best places around the world. We are constantly refining our products as we enhance and create new formulations.

There are many raw material suppliers who manufacture inferior products. Also, there are many raw materials coming from China, which allows for manufacturing at lower costs resulting in cheaper prices; however, the quality of the raw materials and therefore the end product is poor. Our manufacturers independently test and analyze every raw material sent to us to verify its purity and potency.

Q: Will oncologists work collaboratively with you and your recommendations to use botanical medicine to help heal cancer patients? Do you try to persuade the patient to listen to your recommendations, or do you try to talk to the oncologist directly?

A: I have found some oncologists to be among the most wonderful hard working people I know, and they are often excited to work with me. Several have become good friends. I just wish we could all work with an open mind, free of the stifling closed mindedness of the currently accepted model.

> **"The greatest obstacle to discovery is not ignorance—it is the illusion of knowledge."** ~Daniel J. Boorstin, 1984.

I will ask the patient, "Do you have an oncologist who will converse with me and look at the information?" I don't make assertions to oncologists without providing solid information, solid data.

Unfortunately, frequently, the doctor will say, "I am bound by my practice to give the chemotherapy drug Gemzar (gemcitabine) for pancreatic cancer. It is what I must prescribe. If I don't, I can be held liable if I do something else, and things don't go well." Even though the response rate is only approximately 15 percent, they will only provide Gemzar.

When a patient reaches Stage 4, the doctor sometimes looks a bit past the standard of care, because there isn't any longer a belief in a possible cure, and now they are willing to look outside the box, but not before this late stage.

Q: How does one go about finding highly competent doctors who are open to integrative, complementary cancer treatments and therapies?

A: It is very difficult; one at a time.

Q: Have you or your associates treated patients successfully who were told to 'get their affairs in order' or who were told that if they did not 'engage in chemotherapeutic or radiation treatments,' they would die? In other words, have some of your patients 'beaten the odds?'

A: They beat the odds all the time. To accomplish these goals, I need to obtain crucial data first. I need data about the patient's body, regarding everything they have done therapeutically and regarding everything that may be related to them and their condition. In addition to talking to the patient, I gather much information from tests, about their tumor markers. I also need patients to be compliant, to follow directions. This is critical.

Beating the odds happens with all different kinds of cancer, even pancreatic cancer patients with poor prognoses. We can often get excellent results with

**pancreatic patients where they live many more years,
five to 10 more years, with a great quality of life,
despite the fact they were given three, six or 12 months
to live by their doctors.**

My approach is complex and adaptive in every way. I offer no quick fixes or alternatives. I use all the lenses and toolboxes of the ETMS and it is all in flux.

Q: Are there any types of cancer patients whom you will not work with, or are you open to most types of cancer issues?

A: We work with every type of cancer, both common and uncommon types of cancer, including pediatric situations.

Q: I understand you provide educational, clinical training in the ETMS process to medical doctors, oncologists, naturopaths, and other practitioners so they can create personalized protocols and increase their expertise in diagnostics and therapeutics. Would you like to comment about this program?

A: Education is one of our core programs. I engage in clinical training twice per year. We have a wide range of practitioners, including: oncologists, other medical doctors, nurses, naturopaths, herbalists, nutritionists, acupuncturists, chiropractors, and others who attend. They attend the ETMS program and are trained over two successive weeks.

We also provide ongoing education with webinars and roundtable groups, once per month. We discuss cancer cases in depth. I also send data daily to the group regarding my ongoing research.

Q: I understand you engage in significant continuing research regarding botanical medicine. Would you like to specify where your information comes from that comprises your research database?

A: I spend many hours weekly reviewing and investigating major medical journals, and their updates. I also review Medscape, Pubmed, and numerous conference updates, and information from other current, credible resources.

Q: What is your vision, five or 10 years down the road, regarding the progress of cancer care?

A: Progress is very slow. I actually believe cancer is becoming more virulent and harder to treat. Cancer has been mutated over generations like resistant bacterial infections. Our vitality has diminished, our stress has increased, and we have become more toxic. Even though we have smarter drugs, their efficacy is not as great as the media and the cancer industry conveys to the public. Breakthroughs are scarce.

Unfortunately, with integrative medicine we are crawling along. There is more "lip service" than good progressive work; however, we have made some progress here and there. In the allopathic arena there has been progress with the drug Gleevec, some drugs for renal cell cancer, and HER2neu targeted therapies, but not much more. Some chemotherapy regimens have been improved, but only marginally.

For the most part, sad to say, the failure in treating the majority of cancers well, is prevalent.

Q: Do you have any suggestions for people who were given a serious cancer diagnosis or who learned of a serious recurrence recently as to how to handle heightened emotions and an appropriate approach to making critically important treatment decisions?

A: We need to use our intelligence to look at issues critically. You must give people hope. When there is no hope, people throw in the towel.

Q: Any final thoughts, comments, or pearls of wisdom you would like to impart to readers of this book?

A: Find doctors and healthcare practitioners who are open-minded.

Before you do anything, take a deep breath.

Study the ETMS approach, also known as Mederi Medicine. Understand what it is philosophically and how it embraces the science of healing, and how we maximize the innate capability of the body (the host) to impact the internal terrain of the host. The process comes from relentless commitment, passion, and love.

References, Resources and Attributions from Donald Yance, Jr., C.N., M.H.

The citations below concern Vitamin D, and pertain to the prior question: "Are there certain tests, i.e., blood tests you use and other diagnostic tests, not generally accepted by conventional medicine, that your experience shows can be determinative of the existence of cancer, the progression of cancer, and that leads you to make specific recommendations?"

1) Rose, A. A., Elser, C., Ennis, M., & Goodwin, P. J. (2013). Blood levels of vitamin D and early stage breast cancer prognosis: A systematic review and meta-analysis. *Breast Cancer Res Treat Breast Cancer Research and Treatment, 141*(3), 331-339.

2) Van Loon, K., Owzar, K., & Jiang, C. (2013, June). 25-hydroxyvitamin D levels and survival in patients with advanced pancreatic cancer (APC): Findings from CALGB 80303 (Doctoral dissertation, 2013). *Program and Abstracts of the 2013 American Society of Clinical Oncology Annual Meeting,* abstract 4022

3) Ma, Y., Zhang, P., Wang, F., Yang, J., Liu, Z., & Qin, H. (2011). Association Between Vitamin D and Risk of Colorectal Cancer: A Systematic Review of Prospective Studies. *Journal of Clinical Oncology, 29*(28), 3775-3782.

4) Ng, K., Sargent, D. J., Goldberg, R. M., Meyerhardt, J. A., Green, E. M., Pitot, H. C., . . . Fuchs, C. S. (2011). Vitamin D Status in Patients With Stage IV Colorectal Cancer: Findings From Intergroup Trial N9741. *Journal of Clinical Oncology, 29*(12), 1599-1606.

5) Chowdhury, R., Kunutsor, S., Vitezova, A., Oliver-Williams, C., Chowdhury, S., Kiefte-De-Jong, J. C., . . . Franco, O. H. (2014). Vitamin D and risk of cause specific death: Systematic review and meta-analysis of observational cohort and randomized intervention studies. *Bmj, 348*(Apr01 2).

6) Li, M., Chen, P., Li, J., Chu, R., Xie, D., & Wang, H. (2014). Review: The Impacts of Circulating 25-Hydroxyvitamin D Levels on Cancer Patient Outcomes: A Systematic Review and Meta-Analysis. *The Journal of Clinical Endocrinology & Metabolism, 99*(7), 2327-2336.

DWIGHT MCKEE, M.D.

ABOUT DWIGHT MCKEE, M.D. Dr. McKee's experience in medical research, oncology, nutritional science, immunology, chemistry, and complementary medicine, combined with his international reputation, confirms his distinguished status as one of the most knowledgeable researchers and clinicians in the world.

He received his undergraduate degree from Williams College with honors in chemistry in 1970, and then entered a combined M.D./Ph.D. program at Case Western Reserve University in Cleveland, Ohio, where he completed the first two years of medical school, as well as full graduate studies in pharmacology and one year of research. After changing his interest from laboratory research to clinical medicine, he completed his last two years of medical school at the University of Kentucky, receiving his M.D. degree in 1975. Dr. McKee completed a rotating internship at the Washington Hospital Center in Washington, D.C., and then became associate medical director of Integral Health Services in Putnam, Connecticut.

Over the next 12 years, he studied and practiced nutritional and mind-body medicine, along with a full range of complementary medicine disciplines. Since completing training in medical oncology, hematology, and immunology, Dr. McKee has been involved in the development of integrative cancer care, working to create a synthesis between conventional cancer medicine and alternative/complementary medicine.

In 2003, he became board certified in nutrition by the Certification Board for Nutrition Specialists of the American College of Nutrition, and in 2007 he became Board Certified in Integrative and Holistic Medicine through the American Board of Holistic Medicine. Dr. McKee has been a member of the Internal Medicine staff at Scripps Clinic, and practiced medical oncology and hematology at the San Diego Cancer Center in Vista, California, where he also served as medical director for Sharp Hospice. He served as a consultant for the San Diego Cancer Research Institute from 2001 until 2010.

Since January of 2001, Dr. McKee has served as Scientific Director of Life Plus International in Batesville, Arkansas, and has co-authored a text on interactions between drugs, nutrients, and botanicals, published by Elsevier Science in 2008. In recent years, Dr. McKee has engaged in consultative and corroborative work with physicians, nationally and internationally, to help them craft integrative treatments and therapeutic protocols for their patients' cancer issues. He has also been a keynote speaker at national cancer conferences, leading and presenting discussions pertaining to the latest breakthroughs in integrative cancer care.

Dr. McKee recently co-authored the book, *After Cancer Care: The Definitive Self-Care Guide to Getting and Staying Well for Patients after Cancer*, published by Rodale Books in 2015.

Interview

Q: What impelled you to become seriously involved in medicine and specifically a cancer practice, and then integrative cancer work?

A: I have a childhood memory of being at a doctor's offices and realizing, "This is what I want to do when I grow up." I was often sick as a child and given lots of penicillin shots in the 1950s. In school, I was quite scientifically oriented and on a medical track as long as I can remember.

At Case Western Reserve University, I was exposed to clinical medicine programs early on. From this experience, I became more interested in clinical medicine and less interested in research. Between 1976 and 1979, I worked as the Associate Medical Director at a clinic in Connecticut called Integral Health Services. It was the first integrative medical clinic on the East Coast, and offered many alternative therapies and health-oriented concepts such as: nutrition, mind-body medicine, yoga, ayurveda, homeopathy, psychotherapy, and other modalities. It provided me with a solid grounding in many novel disciplines and as a result I became board certified in integrative and holistic medicine (American Board of Integrative and Holistic Medicine).

Throughout this time, I was eating very healthy foods and recognized that my chronic health problems were improving. In those days, the medical model viewed the body as a machine, such that when it would break down, a spectrum of symptoms would tell you what kind of breakdown you had and you would then take certain drugs and/or have surgery to deal with the problem.

Nutrition was viewed solely as fuel. It did not matter what the food consisted of. That was the paradigm in those days.

At this time, I also became affiliated with Dr. William Donald Kelly, a dentist who was also a very bright medical intuitive. Dr. Kelly gave his patients huge numbers of supplements as part of his program. Suddenly, I began treating a lot of cancer patients. I was Dr. Kelly's first medical director. He called his program "Metabolic Medicine."

From 1979 to 1985, I worked with various integrative cancer clinics. I organized a clinic at a hospital in Southern California. I also worked at the American International Hospital, the predecessor of the Cancer Treatment Centers of America and worked with a well-known, innovative cancer doctor, Dr. Emanuel Revici in New York City.

In 1988, I decided to pursue a new path to obtain training to become a medical oncologist, despite the fact I was now 13 years out of medical school. I had adopted an inquisitive attitude, to dig deeper, to figure out how and why things work, how they are done, and what might make them work better.

First, I returned to hospital-based post-graduate training at Los Angeles County Hospital and then Santa Clara Valley Medical Center, as well as Stanford University. After becoming board certified in internal medicine, I completed a three-year fellowship in Hematology and Oncology at Scripps Clinic in La Jolla. I also became a visiting scientist at the Scripps Research Institute Immunology Division for two years where I pursued advanced studies in immunology and performed laboratory research in tumor immunology.

From these experiences, I learned that oncologists are too protocol driven. They are much too dogmatic and empirical in their therapeutic approaches, applying results of large randomized clinical trials in a given tumor "type" rather than trying to understand the individual with the disease. I decided I needed to be in control of the whole treatment plan.

Q. President Nixon declared "war" on cancer in 1971. Since that time, the statistics do not seem to support the proposition that we are "winning" the war on cancer. Why not?

A: The medical research regulatory system has become overly bloated and dysfunctional.

It was designed to protect patients, but it has ended up hurting patients. We are not winning the war on cancer.

Not that "war" is necessarily the best approach to dealing with cancer. I think we would do better by studying and learning from cancer, than by waging war on it. What is it telling us about our biology, our environment, our diets, our food supply, our stressors, our society? I believe we could make much more progress if the scientific knowledge was rapidly implemented and integrated.

There is progress in research but it transfers very slowly to clinical practice. Clinical practices are controlled by administrators and financial people who strive for the greatest return on financial investments, which essentially drives oncological practices.

These private oncology practices are the kind at which I practiced during the 1990s. They have been bought by hospitals and large groups like U.S. Oncology Network or Indian Cooperative Oncology Network (ICON). They practice by algorithm.

When I practiced oncology, the bulk of an oncologist's practice and profit was from chemotherapy. Doctors would buy the drugs at low wholesale prices and get reimbursed by Medicare and insurance at high prices. Now, that profit has moved to the large groups and hospitals. The administrators drive the practice of oncologists with requirements about how many patients they need to see, and the fact that they need to generate certain amounts of chemotherapy revenue.

The era of small private practices in oncology, are dwindling. I suggest you read "The Bitter Pill: Why Medical Bills are Killing Us" (*Time Magazine*, 2013), an enlightening story about why medical costs are strangling medicine.

We have made tremendous progress in "the rare cancers." We can cure germ cell tumors, and about half of the lymphomas, as well as a much higher percentage of early stage lymphomas. We have also made excellent strides with chronic myelogenous leukemia with Gleevec (and now 2nd and 3rd generation versions of it), which was the first of what are called "targeted agents".

However, the cure rate is about 12 percent for cancers that have spread beyond their original site when combining radiation and chemotherapy. A large meta-study has shown that chemotherapy alone cures only 3 percent of metastatic cancers, because the chemotherapy responsive cancers such as the one Lance Armstrong had are uncommon.

In Germany, all it takes for a doctor to give an unlicensed drug to a patient that they believe may benefit the patient is to get informed consent and demonstrate that the drug is controlled, pure, and that there is some rationale for giving it. They can give patients new and innovative things much, much easier than here in the United States. Here, cancer has become an industry that only

Big Pharma can play in, because the costs of drug development and drug approval are so high.

> **If a drug does not have a composition of matter patent, then it won't get developed, even if it is the cure for cancer. Natural substances are not patentable under U.S. and European law.**

Q: The term integrative cancer care seems to take on many connotations. What are the most significant distinguishing factors, in practice, which separate strict "standard of care" cancer practices from integrative cancer practices?

A: There is a very broad range of cancer therapies that are done in integrative departments at large cancer centers such as: massage, acupuncture, music therapy and other "soft" therapies. Nine of the 10 top academic cancer centers have integrative departments; some even prescribe a modest program of supplements and vitamins.

Q: Although these therapies can certainly be beneficial, I tend to think of these "soft" therapies, as you put it, as "Integrative Lite." Is that a fair assessment?

A: Yes, that is a good term for it. There is no standard of care, no standardization in integrative cancer therapy. It is very much patient driven. Many centers offer it to grow market share. The oncologists and institutions tolerate it now, more than they used to, but they certainly don't embrace it.

Q: What are the philosophical distinctions between the two concepts?

A: Oncologists are used to multicenter phase 3 randomized trials. The evidence is strong, but the actual results are "nothing to write home about." A two-month incremental median survival improvement is considered a success. They only accept evidence from extremely expensive clinical trials.

On the contrary, when you approach oncologists and state, "We have this great integrative therapy which has had great success," and then specify the fact that a lot of botanicals are used in the protocol, and point out that patients have much better outcomes, the oncologists ask for the evidence. They won't accept evidence generated by wonderful patient experiences and excellent outcomes resulting from clinical practices. They only accept evidence from large randomized multi-center clinical trials.

Q: What about the concept of let's "kill the cancer" versus "building the immune system"?

A: Conventional oncology is an "all-out war on the tumor" philosophy. Alternative cancer therapy is polarized from what is often called the "cut, burn, and poison" philosophy. Alternative therapies want to attack tumors with non-pharmaceuticals and with dosages that may not achieve the best outcomes, depending upon the stage and virulence of the cancer. The alternative adherents strive to "change the terrain" and build up the immune system. Occasionally, that works. With indolent tumors it can work, more so than with an aggressive, fast-growing tumor.

Integrative therapies do both. My career evolution was first alternative, then I trained with the conventional approach, and then I began to integrate the two therapies. I believe we need to use the tools of conventional therapies selectively with the alternative therapies, also selectively.

That is why I became interested in Dr. Nagourney and Dr. Weisenthal's chemosensitivity testing. Let's see if the drug can, at least in the test tube (in a tissue culture system), kill the tumor cells. If it won't work in the test tube, it's not likely to work in the person, unless you have some kind of modifying "Donnie Yance Level of Knowledge" of botanicals or an astute naturopath who has significant knowledge about dealing with resistance mechanisms that tumor cells possess.

Q: How can we get doctors at the large cancer centers, as well as conventional oncologists in general, to become more open to complementary treatments and therapies, in addition to the standard of care?

A: If we can show changes from studies, changes in gene expression due to botanical programs versus control groups we can, hopefully, get recognition and traction.

Q: How can patients find highly competent doctors who offer top-notch integrative cancer care? There are many doctors who claim to be cutting-edge integrative practitioners, but how can patients determine if such assertions are true?

A: By word of mouth and talking to other patients. They are hard to find. You must interview practitioners, and talk to a lot of patients.

Q: What is your opinion about chemotherapy as a treatment in fighting or debulking cancer tumors?

A: Giving patients lower doses, on a more frequent basis, so you don't compromise blood counts.

A metronomic approach (especially if targeted with prior chemosensitivity testing of a fresh tumor biopsy specimen) in most cases, generally given weekly, is the best way to give chemotherapy, in my opinion.

The advantage is, you reduce toxicity and increase the anti-angiogenic effect. Insulin Potentiated Chemotherapy (IPT) has become very popular in the integrative/alternative community, and it is essentially a metronomic approach to giving chemotherapy. We don't really know how much the insulin contributes, as there have not been clinical trials comparing the same chemotherapy drugs in the same doses and schedules given with and without the insulin, and "glucose rescue" used with IPT.

Chemotherapy is a useful tool in certain circumstances; however, it is frequently badly and overly-used.

There is a point where it does more harm than good, but in certain cases it can save your life, for example, if you have metastatic testicular cancer, or an intermediate grade lymphoma. A major weakness with cancer therapies today, is that they don't address cancer stem cells. Chemotherapy kills the daughter cells, but it doesn't kill the cancer stem cells.

There is a very interesting compound called salinomycin, pertaining to cancer stem cells.

There was a team at MIT, which included Dr. Robert Weinberg that engineered a cancer stem cell that had all the characteristics of a stem cell. They studied this engineered cancer stem cell and they used it for a screening of 16,000 different compounds. There were some botanicals that had some activity though they were not very potent. Metformin (a medication used in diabetes) had some activity, but far and away, the most active compound was one derived from a fungus that has been used as an additive to animal feed for over 30 years. It's known as salinomycin.

Dr. Cord Naujokat at the University of Heidelberg in Germany was the first to use salinomycin clinically, with very intriguing results. He published an article entitled "Salinomycin as a Drug for Targeting Human Cancer Stem Cells" in the *Journal of Biomedicine and Biotechnology*, in 2012.

Dr. Mark Rosenberg has had a clinic in Bogota, Columbia where he gave patients salinomycin also with very intriguing results. To my knowledge, the only three groups in the world that use salinomycin are Dr. Rosenberg's group, Dr. Naujokat's in Germany, and one integrative practitioner I know of in Australia. It would be illegal to use this drug in the U.S., because it has not been FDA approved, which would require multiple phases of clinical studies culminating in a large Phase 3 randomized multicenter trial.

Salinomycin could be very helpful with cancer stem cells after obtaining a remission with some combination of surgery, chemotherapy and/or radiation, but there is no "composition of matter patent" for salinomycin. There was a patent approximately 30 years ago, but not anymore.

> **This is an ironic tragedy based upon how our drug approval system is set up, economically and politically. The fact that a composition of matter patent cannot be obtained means there is no interest by drug companies in salinomycin (or non-pharmaceutical agents) as a cancer-fighting compound to inhibit and eliminate cancer stem cells.**

Again, that is because they cannot obtain the financial monopoly as the sole purveyor of the compound and protect the potential for huge profits.

Knocking down the cancer stem cell population would probably reduce the risk of relapse. This is not widely known by the medical establishment. There are a number of botanicals with anti-cancer stem cell activity, and when used together may be fairly potent, but we really need more research in this area.

Q: Do you recommend patients obtain chemosensitivity testing?

A: I think these tests are tremendously valuable.

> **Yes, the gold standard, in my opinion, is what Dr. Nagourney and Dr. Weisenthal do.**

My ability to make tremendous differences with advanced stage cancer patients took a quantum leap when I had patients engage in the kind of chemosensitivity testing performed in labs operated by Dr. Nagourney and Dr. Weisenthal, which are fundamentally the same, with minor differences.

Q: What is your opinion about genomic testing?

A: The cancer world is way too excited about genomic testing.

> **There are abnormalities in the genome in cancer, but there is also good evidence that abnormalities also take place in the cytoplasm and mitochondria.**

If you transplant the nucleus of a cancer cell into the cytoplasm of a healthy cell, that cell becomes healthy. If you transplant a healthy nucleus into a cytoplasm of a cancer cell, it remains cancerous. So, the cytoplasm trumps the nucleus in those experiments. I think both are important.

The problem is, we have been focused only upon the DNA abnormalities in the cell nucleus with chemotherapy and radiation research. However, everything we talk about in metabolics is relevant to what is going on in the cytoplasm and in the tissue microenvironment within tumors. Another thing that has led us down the primrose path clinically is the research focus upon individual cancer cells, as in particular "cell lines," which are cells isolated from human tumors that have been immortalized with a virus. This changes them, and they no longer are the same as the tumor cells from which they were derived. They are more sensitive to many things than real tumor cells in patients.

It is also now readily apparent that there is serious communication between tumor cells and normal "stromal" cells in their microenvironment. The stroma and related vascular activity, as well as infiltrating immune cells, is definitely part of the process. Chemosensitvity testing should also look, seriously, at the stromal tissue, not just cancer cells.

Q: Regarding chemotherapy, are there studies and peer-reviewed medical literature that address the efficacy and safety of using certain vitamins, botanicals and extracts to mitigate toxicity and enhance the effect of chemotherapy? Can you comment on these issues?

A: There are lots of observational studies and suggestive evidence supporting the proposition that there is real benefit and protective activity, enhancing the efficacy of chemo with the use of certain vitamins, botanicals and extracts. Unfortunately, we don't have big studies, because these types of therapies are not patentable; therefore, no one will spend a billion dollars to finance a protracted, large study.

> **I am completely comfortable with the use of specified botanicals, minerals, antioxidants and vitamins concurrently with chemotherapy and radiation therapy and have seen very good results, clinically, in my own practice.**

It is dogma among radiation oncologists that antioxidants will interfere with radiation, and some even say, "Don't eat kale or blueberries during radiation, because they are too strong of an antioxidant." It is true that radiation has its effect on cancer cells partly through an oxidative mechanism with oxygen; you are creating oxygen free radicals and tumors that are low in oxygen which respond less well than those that are well oxygenated.

There is also an oxidative stress mechanism with certain types of chemotherapy. But the evidence that does exist suggests that modest doses of antioxidants and an antioxidant rich diet do not interfere with the anti-tumor effects of radiotherapy and chemotherapy. I do advise patients not to take supplements the day of chemotherapy, with a certain few exceptions. There is also good research evidence that plant derived compounds, such as curcumin, have anti-oxidant effects in healthy cells, but oxidative effects in cancer cells. In other words, they seem to possess a type of "intelligence".

Q: Can fasting help cancer patients?

A: I advise patients to fast the day before, the same day and the day after chemotherapy. Water and tea are OK, but it is essentially a fast.

**The fast appears to cause normal cells to down regulate
their metabolism and hibernate. Cancer cells can't
hibernate. This concept reduces toxicity and comes from
Dr. Valter Longo's work at the University of Southern
California. I know that fasting works based upon my
clinical practice.**

Generally, patients who fast successfully do not get sick, but those who do not fast sometimes become very sick. I've also seen patients get quite sick on their first cycle of chemotherapy, and then fast with the next cycle and do much better, even though it's the same chemotherapy. Patients who are underweight may not be able to tolerate fasting with chemotherapy. Clinical trials are underway to look at fasting with chemotherapy in a systematic way.

Q: Do conventional oncologists approve of certain vitamins, botanicals, and extracts to mitigate toxicity and enhance the effect of chemotherapy?

A: No, for the most part, they don't. They don't want their patients to take anything that may be an antioxidant, and they're very concerned about herb-nutrient-drug interactions, which for the most part are theoretical. A lot more clinical research in this area would be very helpful.

Regarding treatment interventions like chemotherapy, a question that integrative practitioners must assess is whether their patient is being treated by the oncologist with curative or palliative intent. If the patient is being treated with palliative intent, they generally have more freedom to add integrative therapies versus the strict standard of care. If the patient is being treated with curative intent (for instance early stage breast cancer), it's best to work mainly with diet and lifestyle.

Even in the best situations, cure will not be 100 percent, and if integrative therapies that are not accepted by the oncologist, such as vitamins or herbs are added, and the patient relapses or doesn't achieve a complete remission, it's likely that such integrative treatments will be blamed.

Q: Can you address the issue of targeting pathways and how drugs work in this manner, versus how integrative tools target pathways?

A: At the most, drugs have six targets; however, most drugs have only one or two targets. When botanicals are used, strategically, they have a weaker direct effect than chemotherapy, but they also target dozens and sometimes hundreds of targets. Picture metaphorically, the graphic from *Gulliver's Travels*, where the giant is restrained with hundreds of tiny threads. The thin tiny threads, alone, are not particularly strong, but in combination, they can be powerfully effective. That is how I envision the activity of botanicals against tumors.

Q: What kind of testing, blood work, evaluations, and assessments do you think are most important so that cancer doctors may craft comprehensive regimens to offer optimal "personalized" cancer care?

A: Generally, tests to monitor inflammatory markers, angiogenisis markers, hyper-coagulability and other immune system markers are critical.

Along these lines, inflammation is the food for cancer. Ironically, everything we do in conventional cancer therapy creates inflammation. Radiation creates inflammation. Chemotherapy creates inflammation. Surgery creates inflammation. Even immunotherapy creates inflammation. One of the jobs of the integrative physician is to support patients with the goal of reducing inflammation.

For most patients, the following laboratory tests are useful to obtain valuable information, prior to consultation. In specific instances, other tests may be needed on a per case basis:

1) CBC and Blood Chemistry Panel: Numbers outside the normal range may suggest disorders indicating the possible presence of cancer. Low hemoglobin means that tumors are more likely to have low oxygenation, which causes them to become more aggressive and likely to spread.

2) 25-OH Vitamin D: There is demonstrable evidence that a vitamin D deficiency points to a higher risk of certain cancers. For cancer patients, I like to see the blood level of 25-OH vitamin D between 50 and 80 ng/ml. One must be careful, however, with lymphoid malignancies and patients with any co-existing granulomatous disease (e.g., sardoidosis), as they may be vitamin D sensitive, and develop very high 1,25 di-OH vitamin D (the activated form), and subsequent hypercalcemia.

3) Hs-CRP: As a marker for chronic inflammation, this test assists in the identification of subjects with an increased risk of cancer. Inflammation feeds cancer and vice versa. I like to see this value < 1.0, or as close to that as we can get it.

4) HgbA1C: This blood test, used by diabetics to measure their average blood sugar is strongly predictive of cancer development. Diabetics have a higher propensity to cancer. I like to keep this below 5.4 percent in cancer patients. In patients at high risk of relapse, as low as < 5.0 percent. During treatment, it is important to realize that the HgbA1C number assumes a red blood cell lifespan of 120 days, and cancer patients often have a much shorter red blood cell lifespan. Therefore, the HgbA1C number often underestimates their average blood sugar. The value depends upon, both the level of blood glucose, and the time that the hemoglobin (in red blood cells) is exposed to it.

5) IGF-1: Higher blood levels of IGF-1 indicate a higher risk and link to various cancers.

6) DHEA-s: High serum levels may be indicative of adrenal gland cancers and certain other cancers. We usually don't try to raise DHEA in hormone-driven cancers such as ER+ breast cancer or prostate cancer, as it can be made into either androgens or estrogens, and is somewhat unpredictable in this regard.

7) Fibrinogen (activity): High plasma fibrinogen levels from this test represent the real possibility of tumor invasion and metastases. Higher fibrinogen levels also reflect chronic inflammation. I like to keep this value below 300 if possible. An enzyme called lumbrokinase is useful in lowering it, and also reducing the risk of blood clots, which is always an elevated risk in cancer patients. Lumbrokinase (and nattokinase) may also help digest a fibrin sheath that tumors coat themselves with, as one mechanism to hide from the immune system. This may be particularly important with the new immunotherapies.

8) Quantitative D-dimer (if tumor is present): This is a prognostic biomarker associated with poor survival in the overall cancer population. High levels can be predictive of the occurrence of venous thromboembolism in cancer patients. Lumbrokinase, as part of a comprehensive program, can often help to lower it.

9) Homocysteine: Elevated levels of homocysteine (an amino acid) are indicative of poor methylation, a process which is often weak in cancer patients, and may predispose to developing certain cancers.

10) Serum copper: High copper levels have been found in many types of cancers. Copper is an important cofactor for angiogenesis.

11) Zinc: Zinc tests can indicate zinc deficiency, which can cause an impaired immune function. I like to get the zinc to high normal, and copper to low normal in people with cancer challenges.

12) Ceruloplasmin: Ceruloplasmin (a protein produced by the liver that binds copper for transport in the blood) is significantly elevated in advanced cancers.

13) Selenium: Studies show that low levels of selenium are associated with a higher risk of cancer death.

14) Serum retinol (Vitamin A): Studies have shown the capacity of vitamin A to reduce carcinogenesis. I like to get this to high normal range in patients with squamous cancers, where vitamin A has significant differentiating activity (helps cells become more normal).

15) Serum galectin-3 level (Labcorp): Elevated levels have been linked to the development of several different cancers as well as cancer metastasis. Modified citrus pectin works against galectin 3 (athough it won't lower the levels), and discourages metastases.

16) Exatest: Sublingual epithelial cell scraping for intracellular, magnesium. Magnesium deficiency seems to promote carcinogenesis; thus the test can indicate whether magnesium supplementation would be recommended to inhibit carcinogenesis.

In breast and prostate cancer cases, add:

1) Serum estradiol: High levels of estradiol are associated with increased risk of post-menopausal breast cancer.

2) Estrone sulfate: It is speculated that a major source of estrogen in breast cancer cells may be the conversion of estrone sulfate to estrone by the enzyme estrone sulfase. Thus, inhibitors of estrone sulfate may have the potential for the treatment of estrogen dependent breast cancers. Therefore, the test assessing the prevalence of estrone sulfate can be very important.

3) Total and free testosterone: These tests can help determine risks associated with prostate cancer patients.

4) Prolactin: This is a hormone produced by the pituitary gland. Its primary role is to help initiate and maintain breast milk production in pregnant and nursing women. A high level may indicate the existence of tumors that produce and release prolactin, including the possibility of other tumors. Prolactin can also stimulate both breast and prostate cancers, so keeping it low in these cancer types is useful.

5) TSH: Free T3, free T4, reverse T3: These tests can indicate potential disorders and possible cancers of the thyroid and pituitary gland.

Q: Are these specific tests different from those offered by doctors engaged in strict standard of care practices?

A: Yes, very much so.

Q: I have heard integrative and alternative doctors say, "Biology is not destiny" or "Genetics are not your destiny." What does this mean?

A: There are important identical twin studies. In the largest study ever conducted among identical twins, which means they share 100 percent of their genes, published in the *New England Journal of Medicine* in July, 2000, researchers found that for all cancers combined, the twins developed the same cancer only about 10 percent of the time.

This demonstrates that the onset of cancer is due primarily to epigenetics, i.e., diet, lifestyle conditions, exposures, and issues encountered throughout people's lives. Some scientists even believe hereditary causes of cancer are closer to 5 or 10 percent.

The way you live your life can significantly change your genome and impact whether you get cancer or not, in contrast to the age-old belief that most cancers are inherited. In brief, most cancer is made, not born.

Q: That's a compelling study. Any other thoughts on this issue?

A: Yes. Looking at the BRCA1 and BRCA2 genes, I strongly believe that if you observed twins who had the BRCA1 or BRCA2 mutations, and one twin lived a strict healthy lifestyle, versus the other twin who lived a junk food and unhealthy lifestyle, that twin would get breast cancer; the other one would not.

When you study the work of the renowned geneticist, Mary-Claire King, Ph.D., you realize that she looked at women born before 1940, with a strong genetic risk, and it was determined that they had a 24 percent risk of developing cancer by the age of 50. Those women born after 1940, with the same genetic risk, showed a 67 percent risk of getting cancer. This strongly suggests that changes in the food supply (more processed food, sugar-laden foods, institutionally fed animals) that have occurred more during modern times, post-World War II, including environmental changes and one's overall lifestyle, play an important role in increasing the chances of women with BRCA mutations to develop breast cancer.

Q: Some people say, "I tried integrative or alternative medicine and it did not work." How might you respond to this statement?

A: There is no exact standard of care in integrative or alternative medicine. There is not a specific standard or best type that applies to different situations. There are distinctions between different types of integrative and alternative medicine treatments. People need to keep looking until they find a system/ practitioner that works for them.

Q: What is your opinion about the efficacy and safety of complementary treatments and therapies? First, what about dietary recommendations?

A: There is much difference of opinion on this issue. I think different people have different nutritional needs based on their genetic background, their health status, the environment they live in, the work they are doing, and other factors.

Whether you should be vegan, paleo, raw food or something else is very individualistic. They can all work for different people.

Clearly, I strongly suggest the avoidance of processed food, a high sugar diet and an oxidized fat diet. I do encourage a whole-foods, organically grown approach to eating. You certainly can't rely on what the food industry is producing. You must find the "blend" of foods that resonates for you. I know some practitioners are ideologically wedded to their diets. Flexibility is, in my experience, a better approach. At the same time, if a patient is anemic or underweight, they may need some red meat, at least for a while, but they should find pasture raised and organic beef or goat.

Q: Supplementation?

A: Vitamins, botanicals, extracts and other types of supplements can be very effective.

You need to have a scientific understanding of what kinds to prescribe, the specific dosage levels, including when and how to customize a protocol tailored to every patient. You need to have a sophisticated understanding about how various supplements affect the body in general, how they influence cancer tumors, and how they impact the overall wellbeing of the patient.

In addition to supplementation, there is a whole world of "off-label drugs" that are not specifically known as cancer drugs, but many of them are useful in treating cancer. Metformin, the most commonly used drug for type II diabetes, is one of them.

Q: What about mind-body and stress reduction therapies?

A: Anybody with cancer will have psychological issues. I often recommend that patients should speak with someone knowledgeable in this area, in their geographic region. There are many different mind-body and stress reduction therapies that may help patients deal with cancer—and improving stress management has been shown to lead to better survival in cancer.

One example concerns an 11-year study of a stress management technique known as "progressive muscle relaxation" with breast cancer patients, at high risk of relapse, at the James Cancer Center of Ohio State University. The study found that regular practice of this technique reduced the risk of dying of breast cancer by 56 percent. (See researchnews.osu.edu/archive/cancrecurrence.) There is no reason to expect that these benefits would be confined to a single cancer type. Progressive muscle relaxation is a technique taken from Hatha Yoga, often taught at the end of a yoga class. When the study was looked at for all causes of death, those who regularly practiced PMR versus those who didn't had a 68 percent overall reduced risk of dying. This is a bigger effect than adjuvant chemotherapy and hormonal therapy combined.

There are also many other relaxation and stress management techniques, for example, meditation, yoga, tai chi, qi gong, heart math and other types of biofeedback, that have not been studied in relation to cancer outcomes, but which are very likely beneficial.

I have also learned that patients who are motivated by something unfinished in their life, like raising a child, or those with a goal to achieve an unfinished work, do much better than those who are motivated primarily by fear of dying. Unfortunately, many people involved in treatments are motivated by the fear of dying versus a drive to accomplish specific things. Dr. Bernie Siegel talks about these issues in his books.

Additionally, if you tell people with metastatic cancers that they will get better with any type of therapy, 10 percent will achieve dramatic durable remissions with widely divergent kinds of therapies. There is definitely a mind-body component with cancer.

Q: Is exercise helpful?

A: Yes, exercise in many forms can be very helpful. It can also be very helpful during chemotherapy. Dr. Keith Block has had excellent results in this regard, encouraging his patients to exercise, even while chemo-therapy is being delivered, and achieving significant reductions in side effects. In fact, it is now being recognized, even in mainstream oncology, that exercise is the ONLY intervention that mitigates cancer treatment induced fatigue.

Q: What about the concept of maintenance? How can someone who is in remission optimize his or her chances of preventing a recurrence?

A: With Stage 4 metastatic patients who have achieved complete responses (complete disappearance of tumors on scans, and normal tumor markers), copper chelation, taken over three years (oral dosing, taken daily) is a powerful strategy to prevent relapse. Let me give you some background.

Copper is believed to be the switch that turns on the angiogenesis process in tumor cells. It has been observed that abnormally high serum copper levels are found in patients with many types of progressive tumors.

According to the University of Michigan Oncology Journal, many studies have shown copper to be an obligatory cofactor in the process of angiogen-esis. Growth factors in angiogenesis require binding to copper in order to function properly. As Dr. Steven Brem states in his research at the Moffitt Cancer Center, "Copper-binding molecules (ceruloplasmin, heparin, and the tripeptide glycyl-histadyl-lysine) are non-angiogenic when free of copper, but they become angiogenic when bound to copper."

On January 21, 2000, the University of Michigan reported that researchers had successfully stopped the growth and spread of cancer by depriving the tumors of the copper supply they need to form new blood vessels. This study was done with a small group of patients with advanced cancer. Researchers used an inexpensive compound called ammonium tetrathiomolybdate (TM) a molecule combining four sulfur-hydrogen groups bound to an atom of the mineral molybdenum, to lower the ceruloplasmin (CP) levels (the major copper binding protein in blood) in patients with cancer.

Because TM is not patentable, although available through compounding pharmacies, it has not been further developed by the cancer pharmaceutical industry. However, a newer molecule called choline tetrathiomolybdate has been patented, and is in clinical trials in the E.U. and the U.S., as a treatment for Wilson's disease. If it is eventually approved in the U.S. for Wilson's disease, it could be used as "off label" for cancer patients as well.

Let me give you more explanation about the strategic focus of how to use tetrathiomolybdate (TM). The goal of copper chelation with TM as an antiangiogenic strategy is to lower ceruloplasmin (CP) to the target level, which is 15 to 20 percent of the baseline level, and keep it at that level for at least 90 days, to see if the strategy will halt tumor growth. At this point, if any stabilization of tumor growth has occurred it should become apparent from scans taken at the 90-day point after reaching the target CP and compared to scans done after another two to three months (longer for tumors that have historically been slow growing). This is a long-term strategy, though, and these levels should remain low to prevent new blood vessels from growing.

I have found TM to be most effective when applied in the No Evidence of Disease (NED) setting. For this strategy to work, CP needs to be maintained in the target range (I now generally aim for 10 mg/dl, with a range of 7-15 mg/dl if the blood counts tolerate that), or the lowest level that maintains acceptable blood counts.

When tumors are large enough to be seen on scans, these tumors are already angiogenic. Depriving them of the copper dependent angiogenesis growth factors slows them down for a while, but eventually most of them progress— presumably by learning to use angiogenesis growth factors that are not copper dependent. However, with very small tumor cell colonies (<2 cubic mm), it is much more difficult for them to develop angiogenesis, which they must have to grow larger than this size, without the function of the half dozen copper dependent angiogenesis growth factors.

My clinical experience has shown that if these sub-angiogenic (tiny) tumor colonies (which we can't see with scans, but can only presume the presence of) are deprived of the copper dependent angiogenesis growth factors, by maintaining a subclinical level of copper deficiency with TM for three years, that subsequent relapse is very rare, even after TM is discontinued.

Essentially, the copper chelation prevents them from attaining angiogenesis. It engenders tumor dormancy and probably impacts cancer stem cells.

Q: Can patients go back to living their life as they did, prior to their cancer diagnosis, or should they make serious lifestyle changes?

A: I have often told patients, "Cancer can bring about the best lifestyle choices you will ever make." Cancer patients must make serious lifestyle changes to recover and they must maintain those changes, long-term. Otherwise, they will recreate an internal biochemical terrain that may be conducive to the recurrence of cancer.

Q: I understand, during your practice, you reported some wonderful outcomes with late stage cancer patients who had recurrent or meta-static cancer issues, including terminal cancer diagnoses and people who had begun hospice care. What has brought about these wonderful outcomes? Is it about the treatments, the sophistication of the doctor, or the individual's "fight" and will to live?

A: I would attribute successful outcomes to all of the above or a combination of many of the above. We can cure Stage 4 cancer, but not predictably or reliably. I will say moderation does not work when you are dealing with advanced stages of cancer. It takes a serious, committed effort on the part of the patient, family, and health care team.

Q: What is your vision, five or 10 years down the road, regarding the progress of cancer care?

A: I would love to see a major global cancer center where patients could have access to all types of treatments and technologies. There is good research occurring that is not translated in both the conventional and alternative worlds. There are also a lot of good things happening in the integrative/alternative world that are not being studied. It takes money.

> **When I started doing some of these things in the 1970s it was called cancer quackery, but now it is called integrative cancer therapy. Unfortunately, clearly, only a minority of oncologists accept real integrative cancer therapy.**

At the same time, I think the progress with the new immunotherapies in mainstream oncology is very exciting. These include what are called "checkpoint inhibitors", which are monoclonal antibodies which block the ways tumors evade the immune system, allowing a vigorous immune response which can result in complete remissions—and when these occur they last a long time— they may represent cures, but we don't know yet, because the therapies are relatively new.

There are also engineered T-cells, adoptive transfer of immune cells (isolated from tumors and then grown in the laboratory and re-infused to the patient), tumor vaccines, and monoclonal antibodies which target tumor cells themselves. These therapies are showing promise in virtually all types of cancer, rather than just melanoma (for which many of them were originally developed) and kidney cancer, the two types that have traditionally been known to respond, to some degree, to various immunotherapies.

> **I believe we are in the early phases of a paradigm shift, from the age of chemotherapy to the age of immunotherapy.**

The other thing that I believe is very exciting about the development of the new immunotherapies in oncology, is that we have strong anecdotal evidence that "support" with nutrients, diet, and botanicals may be highly synergistic with these new therapies. The monoclonal antibodies aren't metabolized in the liver at all, so many of the concerns about supplements and herbs interacting/interfering with metabolism of chemotherapy drugs go away.

The anecdotal evidence concerns four patients of Donnie Yance, on his full ETMS protocols (intense individualized combinations of diet, medicinal smoothies, individualized botanical tincture blends, herb tea blends, and many supplements of both botanical extracts and nutrients) who went into four different checkpoint inhibitor clinical trials (at Donnie's urging), and all four of them turned out to be the ONLY patients in each of the trials (of 30 to 40 patients each) who achieved a complete response (this means that all evidence of tumors everywhere in the body disappeared completely). Some of the patients told the clinical trial director what they had been doing, but several were afraid to disclose it for fear of disapproval. If these early observations pan out, we may see an oncology environment in which the young oncologists who grew up with these new immune-therapies will eventually recognize that their patients on integrative protocols actually do better, and will welcome and even recommend them—hospitals and cancer centers might even be hiring herbalists—rather than fighting against herbs and supplements as their predecessors did in the age of chemotherapy.

Q: Do you have any golden nuggets or pearls of wisdom that you might impart to people who have just been diagnosed with a serious cancer challenge or who have recently been informed that they are facing a serious recurrent cancer issue?

A: Don't panic; don't be swept up in the psychological emergency of a cancer diagnosis. The cancer has been there for a very long time, based upon our knowledge of cancer biology. There are only a handful of cancer types (small cell lung cancer, lymphoblastic lymphoma, Burkitts lymphoma) that grow so fast that treatment needs to be started very soon after the diagnosis is made.

> **Spend time educating yourself. Find a practitioner who inspires confidence in you. Talk to other patients who have had good outcomes with the practitioner. Find a practitioner who has done good work, and brought about excellent outcomes with integrative work. Word of mouth is probably your best guide.**

Get yourself in good shape prior to conventional treatments.

> **Don't spend too much time on the web. There is much confusing and conflicting information on the Internet.**

Unless you know someone with expertise to help you separate the wheat from the chaff, you can get totally lost, confused and stressed. There are over a million websites that are thinly disguised marketing sites for cancer remedies, some of which may be useful, but many are not.

Q: Do you have any final thoughts?

A: As a society, as a culture, the whole idea of a war on cancer is misguided. When we struggle against cancer, we create pain and fear. We don't recognize that it is a deep mystery and very connected to life itself. It is sort of a perversion of life, the shadow side of life's biologic processes.

It is possible to die of cancer and to have been healed on many levels. We should not equate death from cancer as a failure. When you drop dead of a heart attack, you don't get to say goodbye to anybody, nor do you have the chance to resolve issues. You don't get to tell your estranged brother or your spouse or child or parent that you love them.

When people recover from cancer, their relationships are better, their lives are better. Sometimes it takes cancer to get out of a bad marriage or a bad job and then you can embark upon things that are much more fulfilling.

Viewing cancer as a messenger or as a teacher, rather than as an enemy, can be useful on many levels. There is a role for taking on the warrior persona at a certain point, but it is better if you can evolve beyond that to become a scholar.

Assess how and what this disease process has opened you up to, in your life. You can learn a lot from cancer, and really improve your life. Healing your life, and the lives of your loved ones is a transformational experience, which the challenge of cancer offers.

PART THREE

83 Critical Questions to Ask
Before Hiring Your Cancer Doctor

About Part Three The third section of this book is comprised of a number of useful, focused, and critical questions cancer patients should consider asking their prospective doctors and healthcare practitioners, prior to hiring them.

Frequently, many people become paralyzed with fear upon hearing a cancer diagnosis and do not know what to say to practitioners, or what to inquire about. The multitude of inquiries, specified below, may help cancer patients compile a set of important "customized" questions, so that they can learn more about recommended treatments, therapies, and issues related to their cancer situation.

Imperative Consideration: Inquire about the doctor's or healthcare professional's background, knowledge and experience, and the nature of his or her practice. You need to know that they are top notch; that they are highly credentialed, respected and deeply experienced regarding your particular cancer issue.

It's important that your doctor listens to your concerns and questions, and respects your interest in being an informed patient. If the doctor or healthcare practitioner lacks compassion, he or she is probably not a good choice.

It's YOUR Life. Get answers that YOU are comfortable with before choosing a healthcare professional.

83 CRITICAL QUESTIONS

Treatments, Efficacy, Experience and Safety

1. Do you treat cancer patients, predominantly, in your practice?

2. Specifically, what kind of cancer do I have?

3. What stage and/or grade is my cancer and what does that mean?

4. Can Stage 1 or Stage 2 become Stage 3 or Stage 4?

5. If so, how long might it take to become Stage 3 or Stage 4?

6. If I am Stage 3 or Stage 4, can I still live many more years with a healthy quality of life?

7. What treatment options do you recommend and why?

8. What have been the results of each of these treatments with my type of cancer?

9. Is there evidence based on recent or past studies, or your experiences with other patients like me, indicating the potential efficacy of the treatments you recommend?

10. Are there scientific articles written about these studies or trials that you can give me to read and study?

11. Generally, what do these articles say regarding these treatments?

12. Who sponsored and financed these studies?

13. Have the results of the studies been definitive or are they somewhat ambiguous?

14. Are there any studies, or is there any medical literature, that contradicts or questions the effectiveness of these recommended treatments?

15. Is the goal of the treatment(s) you recommend:

    - to cure me?

    - to control the cancer?

    - to slow the progression?

    - palliative?

    - to bring about some other objective?

16. Are there any side effects associated with these treatments?

17. If so, what can I do to mitigate potential side effects, from a conventional or alternative perspective?

18. Do you have experience with non-pharmaceutical agents or pharmaceutical drugs that may lessen side effects?

19. How will my quality of life be affected by the treatments?

20. What are the possible or probable short-term and long-term effects on my health and will I be able to function normally after my treatments?

21. Is it possible that my type of cancer may spread as a result of the treatments?

22. Can secondary or future cancers be spawned as a result of the treatments?

23. What are the overall risks and benefits associated with the treatments you recommend?

24. What treatments or therapies would you prescribe for yourself or a loved one if you were in my situation?

25. Have you ever been wrong, either too optimistic or too pessimistic, in your prognosis with any of your patients?

26. What is the average time for there to be a positive response, more specifically, a good, beneficial response for me?

27. Can you define your idea of this response—what might it look like for me?

28. If I have a good response to treatments, does this correlate with cancer-free survival and healthy longevity?

29. If I have a poor response to treatments, what will we do next?

30. How long will my treatments last?

31. How often are the treatments required?

32. Will treatments occur in a hospital, clinic, your office, some other place or at my home?

33. Will I have contact with you or members of your staff—or someone else during my treatments?

34. If I have questions, may I contact and reach you directly?

35. What is your office protocol for returning telephone calls?

36. Do you return phone calls in a timely manner?

37. What is your best method of communicating with me when my results are either positive or negative?

38. May I share with you the way I prefer to receive news about my test results or other communications from you—and will you and your office staff follow my wishes?

39. How will my progress be monitored over time?

40. What kinds of tests do you recommend to assess my progress?

41. How many people have you treated with my diagnosis?

42. What is your prognosis for my type of cancer and how do you come to this conclusion?

43. How soon should we begin treatments?

44. Am I eligible to wait a few weeks before I begin treatments?

45. What if I choose to refrain from engaging in some of your recommended treatments?

46. What else do I need to know from you about my situation?

47. May I tell you what else you need to know about me and my emotions and attitudes toward my situation and your role as a healer?

Integrative/Alternative Care

48. Do you have much knowledge about integrative cancer care?

49. What is your definition of integrative cancer care?

50. Will you be open to complementary or alternative treatments and therapies?

51. Are you open to my working collaboratively with an expert in complementary or alternative treatments and therapies?

52. Have you ever worked with patients who wanted to implement both conventional and complementary or alternative treatment options?

53. Ask this question if the provider is an integrative or alternative practitioner: Do you continue to study emerging scientific evidence and treatments related to nutritional, botanical, vitamin, exercise, mind-body, and/or other unconventional treatments and therapies?

54. Are you familiar with different types of diagnostic blood work, tumor marker tests, and other ways to evaluate my situation and monitor my progress, that may not be used by conventional healthcare practitioners? If not, are you open to my obtaining other diagnostic bloodwork that may be helpful to a complimentary practioner?

55. Ask this question if the provider is an integrative or alternative practitioner: Do you study and understand how alternative treatments and therapies may impact conventional treatments and therapies?

56. Do you see each patient as an individual and customize a "personalized" and highly specific protocol, or do you view patients generically and recommend a "one size fits all" approach?

57. Is there anything I can do on my own, and in my daily life, to enhance my immune system and/or fight the cancer?

Clinical Trials

58. What is a clinical trial?

59. Who is sponsoring the clinical trial?

60. How is it funded?

61. Is there any cost to the trial?

62. Will I be paid for participating?

63. Will I be receiving a new or experimental treatment or a placebo?

64. What are the goals of the trial?

65. How long in duration is the trial?

66. What are the potential benefits and risks of the trial?

67. Can I drop out of the trial at any time?

68. Who will be my doctor and/or who will be monitoring my progress during the trial?

69. Will I be permitted to include any complementary or alternative treatments during the trial?

70. Will you please explain all legal and medical issues and aspects of this clinical trial and how they might affect me?

Definition of Success

71. What are your definitions of successful treatment, both long-term and short-term?

72. What are your goals, pertaining to your treatment of me?

Financial

73. What is the estimated cost of the treatments and therapies?

74. Do the costs quoted include follow-up care?

75. What portion of the costs do you think my health insurance plan will cover?

Ask Yourself About Your Opinion of the Doctor

76. What is the doctor's or healthcare practitioner's bedside manner?

77. Does he or she have communication skills?

78. Are his or her answers rational and logical?

79. Does he or she seem forthright and honest, or does he or she seem to be telling you what you want to hear?

80. Do your goals and objectives match the doctor's or healthcare practitioner's goals?

81. Does the doctor or healthcare practitioner possess a 'fighting spirit' and/or positive attitude to want to help you beat or control your cancer?

82. Does the doctor or healthcare practitioner seem resigned to statistical prognoses that are applicable to large groups of people that may not be as unique as you?

83. Is the doctor or healthcare practitioner impatient or patient in answering your questions?

ACKNOWLEDGMENTS

There are many people to thank for their unwavering support, encouragement, selflessness and help in bringing this book to fruition. Here are just a few.

First, thank you to my wife, Gail, whose love and support have always been a constant. I have traveled the country attending numerous cancer conferences and have spent innumerable hours working on this book during the past few years. Gail has always been patient and full of encouragement, even when I faced challenges in bringing this book to fruition.

Thank you to my son, Jeremy, who has always supported my efforts knowing that the book had great potential to bring hope and life-saving information to many people.

Thank you to my sister, Wendy (Elizabeth), who has been a wonderful, thoughtful advocate and who has continually cheered me on, with many constructive suggestions, since the inception of this project.

Thank you to my Mom, whose life-long support and belief in me has been boundless. Her unconditional love, forever, has been a source of great strength.

Thank you to my Dad, who passed on 21 years ago, whose unwavering faith in me, and belief in "going for it," has always been a fountain of great inspiration.

Thank you to the five intrepid and internationally renowned cancer specialists who invested much time and effort in providing wonderful, insightful information throughout their personalized chapters. They have spoken with great candor about profound cancer therapies and evidence-based integrative and alternative treatments. Their enormous contributions have proven to be life-saving and, I believe, will continue to be life-saving for many.

Thank you to the 20 courageous, selfless people who shared their journeys, with transparency, about how they **beat cancer** after being told there was no hope. Frequently, they shed many tears when they re-lived their respective stories with me. Their enduring determination and fortitude, the audacity they exhibited in confronting purported death sentences has been tremendously inspirational. They have provided me, and hopefully the readers of this book, with wonderful lessons and guidance about how to live life and how to face great adversity.

Thank you to the consummate professionals, the respective editors, Carl Lennertz and Mary Holden, who have each made valuable contributions pertaining to the style and literacy of this book with their suggestions, editing, and proofreading expertise. Also, a big shout out to Julia Schopick for her help and encouragement, as well.

Thank you to Gwyn Snider for her creativity, patience and diligence. Her work product is self-evident. She has created a wonderful book cover and interior book design.

Thank you to Steve Bennett, my website guru, whose outstanding team has produced a first class website for the book.

Thank you to the many supportive friends who I have met at numerous cancer conferences, nationwide. Your passion for "the cause," your will to live and learn, your authenticity and unconditional love for humanity, has been a constant source of inspiration that has galvanized and transformed me more than you know.

Finally, with heartfelt love, sincere gratitude and appreciation, once again, I sincerely thank everyone mentioned above, and many others who have gone unmentioned. Collectively, you have inspired me to do the seemingly endless work to finish this book and, as I have been told, "Get it done, because many people NEED to read this book!" Let's keep moving forward, together, and make a difference.

Keep the Hope!

Rick Shapiro

ABOUT THE AUTHOR

Rick Shapiro, J.D., is a consultant and researcher in the field of safe, evidence-based, integrative and alternative cancer treatments. The culmination of his work, developed after cancer took his father's life over 20 years ago, is found in his book *Hope Never Dies*. Shapiro is a passionate and tireless advocate who continually seeks to educate the public about proven medical remedies that save lives. He believes there is much to be learned from terminal and late-stage cancer patients who "beat the odds" by living many years past their so-called expiration dates. He is a member of numerous cancer associations and an active member of the Board of Directors of the Annie Appleseed Project, a non-profit organization that educates people about personalized, integrative, and innovative science-based cancer therapies. Shapiro's website is – www.HopeNeverDies.com

CPSIA information can be obtained
at www.ICGtesting.com
Printed in the USA
LVHW08s1033120818
586687LV00013B/1110/P